For Mr.
William Morgan
with my very best
wishes

Dick Ruiz
6/29/15

OPHTHALMOLOGY

at Hermann Hospital
& The University
of Texas, Houston

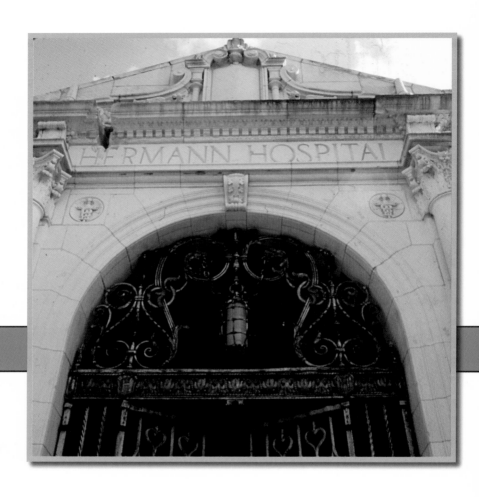

Ophthalmology at Hermann Hospital & The University of Texas, Houston

A PERSONAL PERSPECTIVE

Richard Stranahan Ruiz, MD
& William Henry Kellar, PhD

This paper meets the requirements
of ANSI/NISO Z39.48–1992
(Permanence of Paper).
Binding materials have been
chosen for durability.

Unless otherwise noted, photographs are courtesy of Cizik Eye Clinic.
Photos of historical medical instruments by Maury Jacob and Dan Caplan.

ISBN: 978-0-9846070-0-6

To Yvonne Ruiz

and

To all who believed me

Contents

Illustrations

Foreword

During his internship, Dr. Richard Ruiz decided to specialize in ophthalmology. After completing excellent training in that specialty he returned to his native Houston and its Hermann Hospital to pursue his overarching goal of creating a world-class teaching, research, and patient care eye center. This book is an account of the almost fifty years invested in that effort and of his unusual but outstandingly successful approaches to the structure and support of this unit that capably mixes academic and service functions.

The book is a collaboration of Dr. Ruiz and William H. Kellar, PhD, of the Center for Public History at the University of Houston. Sources are Dr. Ruiz's recollections, various oral histories and interviews recorded and collected over the years, and the files of the Hermann Eye Center Archives. Dr. Ruiz's successful private practice, based in the Hermann Professional Building and the Hermann Hospital, metamorphosed into a group practice, became the core of the Department of Ophthalmology and Visual Science at The University of Texas Medical School at Houston, and adapted to the transformations of the Hermann Hospital from a community hospital with a sizable charity service and some postgraduate teaching, to a major, full-service, tertiary care teaching hospital, and finally to a part of the large, city-wide Memorial Hermann Healthcare System.

The initial chapters cover Dr. Ruiz's background, early life, training, construction of a successful private practice, and his appointment as chief of ophthalmology at Hermann Hospital. Thus, his position was established before the Medical School was started. This has played a key role in his determination and ability to remain simultaneously and steadfastly loyal to, but also independent of, both the hospital and the Medical School. The final chapter outlines how this was creatively accomplished and describes the critical role of the successful Hermann Eye Fund in this effort. The book describes how hard work, persistence, administrative ability, imagination, and courageous entrepreneurial skills have led to the emergence of the world-class eye center visualized by its builder many years ago.

—Cheves M. Smythe, MD, founding dean,
The University of Texas Medical School, Houston

Preface

During the fall of 2006, Richard S. Ruiz, MD, contacted me about helping him write a book that would record the history of the Hermann Eye Center, including the development of the eye service at Hermann Hospital, and the Department of Ophthalmology and Visual Science of The University of Texas Medical School at Houston (UTMS–H), one of the schools of the UT Health Science Center at Houston (UTHSC–H). We agreed on a collaborative effort in which I would conduct the historical research and write an initial draft of the manuscript. This process took about eighteen months to complete. The research included a series of oral history interviews that I conducted with Dr. Ruiz and others who played a role in the history of the Eye Center. In addition, during the late 1980s Ruiz engaged a professional historian, Louis J. Marchiafava, PhD, to interview physicians and nurses who could shed light on the early days at Hermann Hospital. The Marchiafava interviews included sessions with people who had practiced medicine or trained at Hermann Hospital, several of whom are now deceased. These interviews provided an invaluable resource for this project. Other research included both primary and secondary resources found in the collections of the Houston Metropolitan Research Center of the Houston Public Library, the John P. McGovern Historical Collections and Research Center of the Houston Academy of Medicine—Texas Medical Center Library, Special Collections of the University of Houston M. D. Anderson Library, the files of the Hermann Eye Center, and various institutional Web sites on the Internet.

Following the completion of an initial draft, Dr. Ruiz and I began editing and refining the text. During this process, which lasted several months, Ruiz clarified many details and brought his perspective into the book. The final work is comprised of six chapters and an epilogue. The result is a brief overview of the development of eye care in Houston, the role of both Hermann Hospital and later the Department of Ophthalmology and Visual Science of UTMS–H in the creation of the Hermann Eye Center, and the significance of the Hermann Eye Center as a unique model for patient care, education, and research in ophthalmology. It is important to note that Dr. Richard Ruiz served as chief of ophthalmology at Hermann Hospital (later Memorial Hermann–TMC) from 1967 until 2009. In addition, he is the founding director of the Hermann Eye Center and was the first and only chair of the Department of Ophthalmology at the UT Medical School–Houston for the first thirty-seven years of its history. Consequently, Ruiz is the central figure of this history. This book, then, is in part autobiographical and is written primarily from Ruiz's perspective. The book is an important addition to the existing body of knowledge about the evolution of eye care in Houston during the twentieth century, the development of Hermann Hospital/ Memorial Hermann–TMC, the UT Medical School–Houston, and the Texas Medical Center. It should be noted that many of the institutions of the Texas Medical Center have changed names and some have changed affiliations over the years. We have attempted to make note of these changes in the text.

This project would not have been possible without the support and help of many people. First, I must acknowledge Dr. Richard S. Ruiz, who commissioned this project and whose appreciation for history led him to engage the services of Louis J. Marchiafava, twenty years ago, to capture the early history of Hermann Hospital in his interviews. Suzanne Mascola ably transcribed my interviews and, years ago, also did the transcribing for Louis Marchiafava. In addition to conducting interviews in the late 1980s and early 1990s, Marchiafava graciously located lost copies of those transcripts for our use in this project. Much of the information for this history was attained through oral history interviews, and I want to express my gratitude to all who agreed to participate.

Their names and the dates of their interviews are listed in the Note on Sources. Administrative assistance for the project came from Sue McRaney of the Hermann Eye Center, Susan Meng of the Hermann Eye Fund, and Fredi Bleeker Franks of the Richard S. Ruiz, MD Department of Ophthalmology and Visual Science at The University of Texas Medical School at Houston. Historian Kimberly Youngblood and researchers Monica Sanchez and Katy Oliveira used their skills to find key information in Houston area and Internet archives. In addition to her research for this project, Kimberly Youngblood read and commented on several drafts of the manuscript. My colleague from several earlier projects, Elisabeth O'Kane Lipartito, PhD, brought her historical perspective and editorial skills to help improve the manuscript. Thom Lemmons skillfully edited the original text and Mary Ann Jacob applied her artistic talents to create a beautifully designed book. Elizabeth Borst White, Pam Cornell, and Alethea Drexler of the John P. McGovern Historical Collections and Research Center, Houston Academy of Medicine–Texas Medical Center Library helped us find key information and rare photographs in the Center's vast collections. Finally, to all who helped along the way and who must remain anonymous, my deepest thanks.

—William H. Kellar, PhD

Introduction

The Hermann Eye Center has been a prominent aspect of the Memorial Hermann – Texas Medical Center campus for years, predating the merger between the Memorial System and Hermann Hospital. As a contributor to the tripartite mission of research, education, and patient care, the Eye Center has long embodied the vision and ideals that continue to motivate us today. As a research institution, the Eye Center, under Dr. Ruiz's leadership, has made significant contributions to the field of ophthalmology in its basic vision research. Through an educational partnership between The University of Texas Medical School at Houston and Memorial Hermann, Dr. Ruiz and the Eye Center have contributed to the next generation of ophthalmologists, training over 130 residents. In the patient care arena, Dr. Ruiz and the Hermann Eye Center have successfully blended a robust private practice with heroic efforts to meet the ongoing needs of the community, regardless of the patients' ability to pay. This demonstrates the importance of understanding the clinical mission in light of community needs, while developing practices that ensure sustainability for future generations.

The Hermann Eye Fund has facilitated Dr. Ruiz's success by providing financial support from grateful patients that funds indigent care, medical education, and research. Nearly one million dollars in services is provided annually to patients who cannot afford to pay. Through the Hermann Eye Fund, thirteen endowments have been created in the Department of Ophthalmology and Visual Science at the University of Texas Medical School at Houston. In recognition of the department's leadership in ophthalmology, the national organization Research to Prevent Blindness awarded the department in the same year both the prestigious Jules and Doris Stein Professorship and a Career Development Award—the first and only time RPB has granted these two awards in one year to the same institution. The University of Texas paid Dr. Ruiz a singular honor in naming the Department of Ophthalmology at UT–Houston after him.

As ophthalmology continues to move to outpatient surgery settings, the relationship between ophthalmologists and the hospital has evolved. Our role as a Level I trauma center for adult and pediatric trauma ensures that there will always be a need for ophthalmologists to provide trauma care. In addition, many systemic diseases involve the eyes and visual system, including lupus, sarcoidosis, diabetes, thyroid disease, multiple sclerosis, stroke, cardiac disease, infectious diseases, and cancer . Therefore, the ophthalmologist plays an important role in diagnosis and management of our hospital patients. As the Memorial Hermann Healthcare System grows, we will see opportunities for the Eye Center to extend its reach across the system. The commitment to research continues, and there is great opportunity to work collaboratively across specialties in pursuit of new research arenas. I look forward to our continued growth together: the Hermann Eye Center and Memorial Hermann—the legacy of Dr. Ruiz to our community.

—Juanita Romans, CEO
Memorial Hermann Hospital –
Texas Medical Center

OPHTHALMOLOGY
at Hermann Hospital
& The University
of Texas, Houston

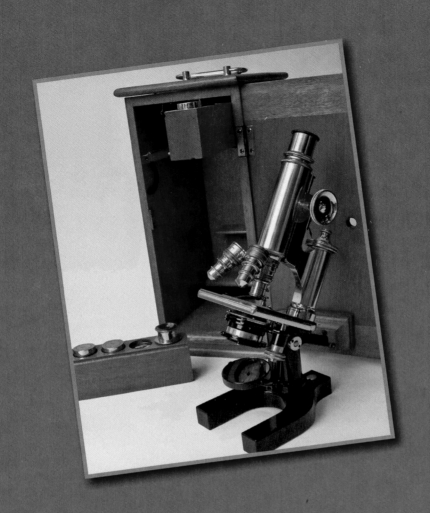

CHAPTER ONE

Early Eye Care in Houston

W ELL, THE MOVE WAS monumental—really monumental," said Dr. Richard S. "Dick" Ruiz, founder of Houston's Hermann Eye Center. On this hot summer day in 2007, Ruiz was seated in his office on the eighteenth floor of the newly constructed Memorial Hermann Medical Plaza, a towering structure with a distinctive crown that stands on the northwest corner of Houston's sprawling Texas Medical Center. In the background, workers scurried busily about, putting the finishing touches on the new facilities. After thirty years on the seventh floor of Memorial Hermann Hospital's Jones Pavilion, all of the files, medical records, furnishings, and ophthalmologic equipment had been packed and moved to the gleaming new building directly across Fannin Street. The move was a culminating moment for the Hermann Eye Center's clinic—renamed the Robert Cizik Eye Clinic in honor of a major benefactor—and for Richard Ruiz, the man who first imagined the possibilities for a world-class eye center in Houston.

The Hermann Eye Center grew out of Ruiz's original ophthalmology practice, his love for teaching, and his desire to be always up-to-date on the latest in research, technology, and treatment related to the eye. The idea for creating the Hermann Eye Center came at a propitious time in the development of medical facilities in Houston. Ruiz first opened his ophthalmology practice in the summer of 1962 in the Hermann Professional Building, directly across the street from Hermann Hospital and the Texas Medical Center (TMC). The Medical Center, established in 1945, was growing rapidly while achieving a level of prominence in the world of medicine, and was an exciting place for a young doctor to begin his medical practice. In 1969, just seven years after Ruiz began seeing patients, officials at The University of Texas announced plans to open a new medical school in the heart of the Texas Medical Center and to affiliate it with Hermann as the primary teaching hospital. Richard Ruiz, who by now had a thriving ophthalmology practice and had been appointed chief of the Ophthalmology Service at Hermann, soon was appointed chair of the Department of Ophthalmology in the new medical school. Thus, the final elements fell into place that enabled Ruiz to seize the opportunity to create a comprehensive eye center. In time, the Hermann Eye Center would become renowned in ophthalmology, patient care, vision research, and education.

The Hermann Eye Center's origins extend well back to the original Hermann Hospital, a significant institution in Houston's medical history. When it first opened in 1925, many welcomed Hermann as Houston's first modern hospital. Prior to its opening, health care in the area had been in transition from the standards and practices of nineteenth-century, frontier medicine to a new era of medical professionalism made evident by improved training and certification for doctors as well as more sanitary hospital conditions. It is interesting to note that from the time the city was established by brothers John Kirby and Augustus C. Allen in 1836, health care had been a major issue that loomed over the growing community. Despite the claims of its founders, Houston's climate was hardly pleasant. The sub-tropical heat and humidity provided a fertile breeding ground for frequent epidemics of cholera, dengue fever, smallpox, and yellow fever. Still, the Allen brothers had chosen a location that had abundant natural resources and was ideally situated for the city's growth as a center for transportation, agriculture, lumber, and cattle. During the twentieth century, that growth would continue as Houston profited in its role as a leading center for oil, petrochemicals, trade, space exploration, medicine, and technology.

While Houston's reputation as a place of economic opportunity grew, so too did its population, including the number of practitioners who provided eye care. Early records indicate that "oculists" and opticians provided most of the eye care for Houston and surrounding areas in the nineteenth century. Evidence suggests that one of the first oculists to advertise in Houston was one J. H. McClintock, whose name appeared in the City Directory in 1879. In 1882, an optician, S. Conradi, advertised that his services were available from his office at 67 Main Street. Within a few years, listings for eye care generally appeared in conjunction with ear care as physicians expanded and combined their practices. In 1889, J. H. McClintock advertised himself as an oculist and aurist. In time, doctors who provided eye care expanded their range of services to other areas of the head and described themselves as eye, ear, nose, and throat (EENT) specialists.

By 1900, eleven listings appeared in the City Directory for EENT care. The level of training and expertise for many of these practitioners before World War I, however, was open to question. The American Medical Association (AMA) began to advocate higher professional standards and improved training around the beginning of the twentieth century. The publication of Abraham Flexner's 1909 study, *Medical Education in the United States and Canada: A Report to the Carnegie Foundation for the Advancement of Teaching*, commonly referred to as the "Flexner Report," added momentum to the push for improved standards of professional medical training. In 1916, ophthalmologists took a major step toward improving professionalism when they became the first medical specialists to establish a board certification program, the American Board for Ophthalmic Examinations. Their goal was to improve ophthalmic practice by creating a certification process that fostered excellence and encouraged continual learning.[1]

Among the earliest of the highly trained, professional ophthalmologists in Houston, two stand out as exceptional. Dr. W. Wallace Ralston, a native Texan, graduated from University of Texas Medical Branch at Galveston (UTMB) in 1899 and served an internship in Galveston at St. Mary's Hospital. Eventually, he studied under some of the finest eye specialists in Europe, including those at the University of Vienna. In 1910, Ralston returned to Texas and set up an ophthalmology practice in Houston. He would rise to prominence, taking leadership roles in a variety of medical societies, including a term as president of the Harris County Medical Society and as the first chief of ophthalmology at Hermann Hospital. Later in 1910, Dr. Everett L. Goar also arrived in Houston and opened a general practice in the Scanlan Building, downtown. Goar grew up in Indiana and studied medicine at Rush Medical College in Chicago. After serving in the Army during World War I, Goar returned to Houston and, later, became acquainted with Dr. Ralston after treating him for pneumonia. Apparently, Ralston encouraged Goar to consider specializing in ophthalmology. Goar soon left to study ophthalmology at the New York Eye and Ear Infirmary (NYEEI opened in 1820 and today is the oldest eye hospital in the United States). He returned to Houston and joined Dr. Ralston in practice in 1921.[2]

In 1922, Drs. Ralston and Goar formed a partnership with Drs. John Foster and Lyle J. Logue, Ear, Nose and Throat (ENT) specialists, and together they built the Houston Eye, Ear, Nose, and Throat Hospital. Dr. Claude C. Cody Jr. joined the group later in the year. The hospital, located on Walker Avenue in the Keystone Building, became one of the primary centers in the city for EENT treatment. Like his mentor, Wallace Ralston, Everett Goar also took a leading role in his profession. Among his many accomplishments, he served as president of the Harris County Medical Society in 1922, as director of the National Society for the Prevention of Blindness from 1952 to 1960, and in 1956 was a co-founder of the Texas Society for the Prevention of Blindness. Goar became chief of the ophthalmology service at Jefferson Davis and Her-

mann Hospitals and served as chairman of the ophthalmology department at Baylor College of Medicine
in Houston. He wrote several widely
used textbooks on ophthalmology,
gaining international renown for
his work. Throughout a career that
spanned almost fifty years, Goar became highly regarded as one of the
leading ophthalmologists in Houston and, indeed, in the nation.[3]

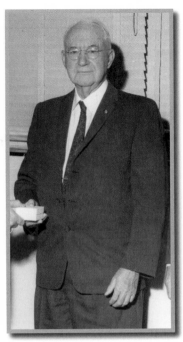

Just as eye care in general—and
the field of ophthalmology in particular—emerged fitfully in Houston, so too did the city's hospitals.
City newspapers indicated some efforts to provide hospitals for Houstonians, but these early attempts

Everett L. Goar, MD, circa 1970.

generally were rudimentary, and often viewed as little more than
"pest houses." As early as 1839, a reference in Houston's *Morning
Star* mentioned "City Hospital" and in 1856, the *Weekly Telegraph*
published a report by Henry Vanderlinden, who was identified as
the Chief Clerk of the Charity Hospital. Of course, one must keep
in mind that until World War I, hospitals held a stigma as places
for the indigent, insane, and terminally ill. Most people turned to
home remedies, folk medicine, or, if they could afford it, family
doctors for their health care. Those who became seriously ill generally found care at home by family members. Later in the century, wealthier patients sometimes sought care in leading medical
centers like Johns Hopkins in Baltimore or the Kellogg Sanitarium in Michigan. Hospital care in Houston took a turn for the
better in 1887 when the Sisters of Charity of the Incarnate Word
opened what would become Houston's first "true" hospital, St.
Joseph's Infirmary. The hospital, which was located in what was
the residential area of LaBranch and Crawford streets, provided

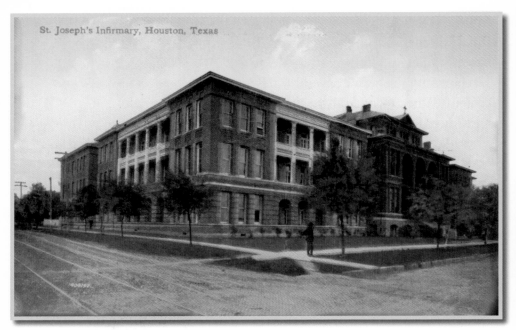

St. Joseph's Hospital, early 1900s. *Courtesy John P. McGovern Historical Collections and Research Center in the Texas Medical Center Library*

high-quality treatment and would be the only institution to sur-vive into the twenty-first century as a major medical center at its downtown location.[4]

During the early years of the twentieth century, several new "pay" hospitals opened to care for Houston's sick. One of the earliest was the Rudisill Sanitarium, located at Smith and Lamar. It was purchased by the Baptists in 1907 and renamed the Baptist Sanitarium (later known as Baptist Memorial Hospital and then Memorial Hospital). The two-story converted house held sev-enteen beds with a staff that included up to ten student nurses. Around this same time, Dr. D. F. Stuart and Dr. S. C. Red opened the Houston Infirmary Sanitarium at Washington Avenue and Tenth Street, offering rooms for the price of one to five dollars "according to location." In 1908, Dr. O. L. Norsworthy opened a hospital on San Jacinto that offered a choice of "ward beds, single rooms with or without a private bath, or two connecting rooms with or without a private bath." The building offered heating by "hot water radiation." By 1911, civic boosters claimed that with the opening of the Southern Pacific Hospital, Houston had become a leading city for providing hospital and medical care for the community. The railroad hospital had electricity and gas, steam heat, and luxurious mattresses. In 1912, Dr. James Greenwood opened a sanitarium for the care of the mentally ill on six acres of land out on Old South Main Street Road. The facility soon added Dr. Marvin L. Graves and Dr. George H. Moody and, along with its twenty employees, provided care for some thirty patients.[5]

By 1914, Houston had a variety of pay-for-treatment hospitals to provide medical care, including basic eye surgery. But later in the year, one of Houston's wealthiest citizens bequeathed a sizeable fortune to improve hospital care primarily for the indigent

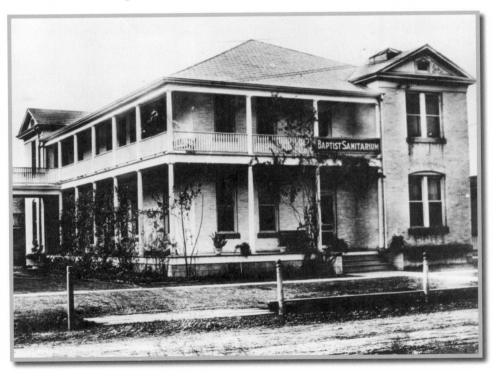

Baptist Sanitarium, 1908—with hitching posts in front—was the forerunner of Memorial Hospital. Courtesy John P. McGovern Historical Collections and Research Center in the Texas Medical Center Library

poor of the city. On October 21, 1914, while being treated for stomach cancer in Baltimore, George H. Hermann died. A frugal bachelor, Hermann, who dearly loved Houston, gave generously during his latter years to improve the community. In June of 1914, he had donated 285 acres of land about four miles south of downtown to establish Hermann Park. In his will, George Hermann left a plot of land downtown and designated $100,000 to build a public charity hospital "for the benefit of the poor, indigent, and infirm residents of the City of Houston."[6]

Houstonians greatly appreciated Hermann's generous gift to the city. Yet, by 1918, Hermann's three executor-trustees had not taken any action to fulfill the conditions of his will. The local newspapers demanded an investigation, while the City of Houston filed a suit demanding an accounting of the estate. The Harris County District Attorney, John H. Crooker, sued, demanding that the trustees be removed. The trustees resigned August 22, 1918, after agreeing that they would "make restitution for the mishandling of the estate."[7]

Nearly four years later, new trustees finally straightened out the affairs of the Hermann Estate, hiring architect Alfred C. Finn of Houston along with the Chicago firm of Berlin and Swern to begin drawing up plans for the hospital. The Harris County Medical Society appointed a committee of doctors to help the trustees in planning the new hospital. The architects performed their task with great care, going so far as to have some of the trustees accompany them to visit several of the newest hospitals in the country to learn the best practices in modern medical design. Construction finally began on the $1.3 million hospital in March 1923.[8]

Hermann Hospital opened for "previews" on National Hospital Day, May 12, 1925. Approximately 35,000 people, including the mayor and city officials, visited the new hospital. And finally, nearly eleven years after George Hermann had died, officials held formal opening ceremonies on July 1, 1925 and began admitting patients on July 13. The new hospital had many features including five operating rooms, an electric kitchen, its own electric light plant, a twenty-ton ice plant, and intercom connections in every room. The head of the American Construction Association claimed, "There is no hospital like it in beauty and efficiency in the South." As historian Marguerite Johnston observed, "Hermann [Hospital] served all Houston and enhanced the practice of medicine, but it did so in ways that George Hermann had not envisioned."[9]

The hospital was located on about twenty acres in what most residents at the time considered "the country," four miles south of downtown, near the Rice Institute. This rustic location created some unique problems for the hospital's administrators. Apparently, the smell of blood and sick patients attracted wolves to the hospital grounds, and the chilling sounds of the animals' howling at night unnerved many of the patients. To deal with the dilemma, administrators had a fence constructed to keep the wolves from getting too close.

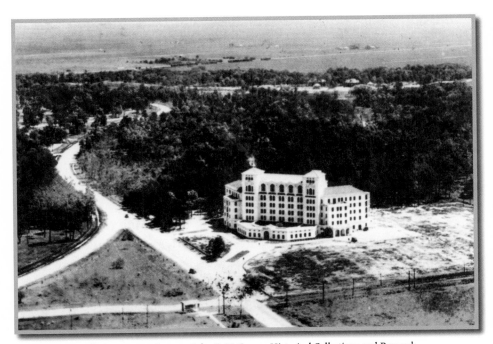

Hermann Hospital, circa 1925. Courtesy John P. McGovern Historical Collections and Research Center in the Texas Medical Center Library

The beautiful Spanish architecture and red tile roof gave the building a distinctive appearance. Naomi S. Foster, Director of Nursing and the Nursing Schools at Hermann, who later compiled an early history of the hospital, wrote that "The hospital building, the only one of its kind in America, was considered a hospital of dreams, a showplace for visitors, and a monument to its benefactor." Visitors entered on the ground floor through a lobby reminiscent of "a grand hotel." Here one found the hospital superintendent's office, the emergency room, an X-ray department, hospital admissions, the business office, medical records, a drug store, a dietician's office, a modern kitchen, and a dining area. For a time, interns' living quarters also were located on this floor. The basement of the hospital contained the morgue, storage areas, and the physical plants and boilers to provide heating, lighting, and ice. Because racial segregation was the rule during this time, rooms for African American patients were located on the first floor, while white patients, both paying and free, were housed in separate wings on the second floor. The patient rooms were built along the outside walls and included ceiling fans, a small toilet facility, and cold drinking water. The fourth floor of the hospital housed obstetrics, pediatrics, and two delivery rooms. The fifth floor held the operating rooms and all surgical support. The hospital had a school of nursing and was the first in the area to offer regular medical internship and residency programs. A list of physicians appointed to Hermann Hospital as of July 1, 1925, included two doctors on the medical staff in ophthalmology: Dr. W. Wallace Ralston, Chairman, and Dr. F. J. Slataper. The medical staff grew from thirty-six to 105 by the end of the year.[10]

Hermann Hospital operated on a strict admissions policy that prohibited three classes of patients from being admitted to the hospital. First were the "incurables," terminally ill patients. The second class included patients suffering from alcoholism, erysipelas, diphtheria, smallpox, typhus, measles, glanders, scarlatina, mumps, whooping cough, cerebrospinal meningitis, scarlet fever, and all other contagious diseases. The third class of inadmis-

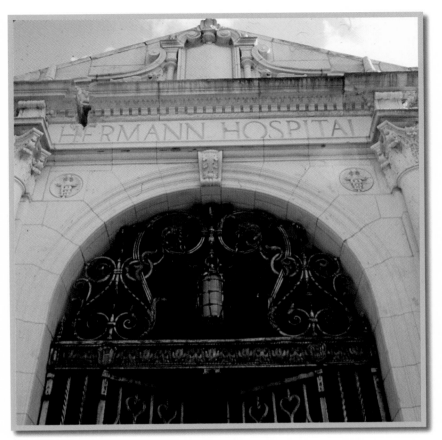

Hermann Hospital's original entrance.

sibles comprised those suffering from any form of insanity. The city and county already had hospitals for these difficult patients and Hermann officials did not wish to replicate those facilities or deplete precious resources when other options were available. Patients who had the means to pay would not be treated for free. The hospital did not begin admitting "paying" patients until 1926. The following year, on May 1, 1927, the board of trustees appointed J. G. Fraidenburg as superintendent. Fraidenburg served as superintendent until 1941. One of his goals was to develop Hermann Hospital so that one day it would be "one of the largest training centers for doctors in the country."[11]

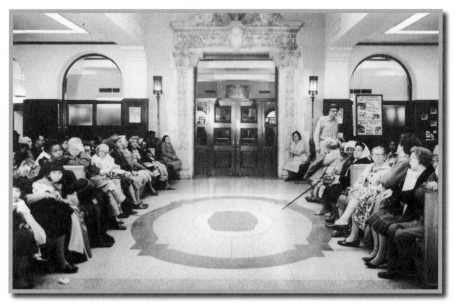

Hermann Hospital—clinic patients' waiting area, circa 1950.

During the next twenty years, as Fraidenburg set out to implement his vision for Hermann, the hospital also began to operate an eye clinic to provide ophthalmic care, mainly for the indigent. Dr. E. L. Goar succeeded Dr. Ralston as chief of the service and essentially ran the program from his downtown office. The Hermann Hospital eye clinic was very small during these years and seems not to have garnered very much support from hospital administrators. During the 1930s, a young high school student, Louis J. Girard, worked as an ophthalmic assistant at Hermann Hospital. Later, Girard attended medical school and in time, would serve as chair of the department of ophthalmology at Baylor College of Medicine in Houston (1956–70). His recollections, as well as those of a number of other doctors who practiced at Hermann, provide a sense of what the hospital was like and particularly how the eye service operated during the first twenty-five years of its history.[12]

Dr. Girard recalled that the eye clinic was located on the ground floor of the hospital. "The clinic in Hermann Hospital at that time was only one examining room. The ophthalmologists would take turns during the six-day week because in those days, everybody worked on Saturday as well. But they would take turns staffing the Hermann Hospital Eye Clinic." Scheduling surgery proved at times to be a major challenge as the surgical theater was very busy and shared by all specialties. The ophthalmologists shared the operating rooms with the other surgeons. The eye surgeons furnished their own instruments because in those days, hospitals didn't own surgical instruments. Each ophthalmologist had to clean and oil the instruments, and then take them to the hospital where they were sterilized and laid out for surgery. Following surgery, the instruments again had to be cleaned, sterilized, and then returned to their special containers. The operating rooms in the old hospital building were on the top, or sixth floor (but called the fifth floor since the entrance level was referred to as the "ground floor"), with large glass windows that overlooked Rice Institute and in the distance, downtown Houston. Girard recalled that "in those days, you have to remember, there was no air conditioning. There were additional windows for ventilation and there were fans going."[13]

Little had changed by the 1940s, when Dr. Elizabeth Crawford began her ophthalmology practice in Houston. She recalled that the Hermann Hospital eye clinic was "a much smaller clinic" than the similar facility at Jefferson Davis Hospital. "And we had almost zero equipment." There was no fund to which the doctors could turn to help purchase equipment at that time. "You just had to request whatever you wanted and probably the department that made the most noise got what little bit of money there was." Dr. Otto L. Zanek, an ophthalmologist who arrived in the late 1940s, stated flatly that the Hermann Hospital eye clinic "was a terrible place to work in" at that time. He recalled the space as "very small and inadequate." Zanek also stated, "I didn't mind seeing patients there, but I hated doing refractions there because the heat was so terrible."[14]

Both Zanek and Crawford remembered Dr. Goar as an excellent administrator. "He was a quiet, sort of terse individual, but he was a very fine ophthalmologist," said Crawford. "I dare say that today, with the exception of [the] retina and one or two things that are newer innovations, that in most offices, patients do not get the care that they did in his office at that time. In a quiet way, he was right on top of everything." Dr. Cecil Crigler, a urologist who came to Hermann during the mid-1940s to organize the urology residency training program, recalled that Goar "was an excellent administrator," and that he excelled "above other people who were doing eye work. They all sent their difficult stuff to him to settle the issue, for the diagnosis. Dr. Goar didn't say a lot, but what he said meant a lot. His administration, I thought, was good and he accomplished, I think, about all he could with the resources he had. And a lot of things that he needed and used in the department, he bought himself—out of his own pocket."[15]

As the years passed, Dr. Goar took the role of senior consultant while Dr. Girard settled in at Baylor. At Hermann Hospital, Dr. Thomas Royce began to take a more active role in the eye service. In 1954, Royce was appointed chief of the ophthalmology service at Hermann. Dr. Crigler noted the changes that began to take place as Dr. Thomas Royce took more responsibility from the aging Dr. Goar during the 1950s. The eye clinic, he recalled, "wasn't much. It more or less met emergencies. And they didn't have the real established rotation of clinic beds and so forth. They'd have days that they would meet various patients there if they had to and if there had to be something done to them surgically, usually [they would be sent] right on down to Dr. Goar's place [Houston Eye, Ear, Nose, and Throat Hospital]." But Royce, who had been the eye physician at the Southern Pacific Hospital, had a different philosophy and became more deeply engaged in the activities of the Hermann eye clinic. "Dr. Royce took the position of a teacher; he took on residents," said Crigler. "Dr. Royce had his offices here in [the Hermann Professional Building] and he carried out the responsibilities that a chief should. Of course, he sat in on our medical education committee every time we met

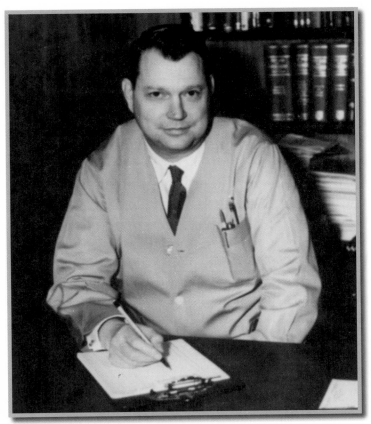

Thomas Royce, MD, Chief of Ophthalmology, Hermann Hospital, 1954-66. Courtesy John P. McGovern Historical Collections and Research Center in the Texas Medical Center Library

and he fulfilled all his responsibilities in his department quite well."[16]

During these years, events taking place beyond the walls of Hermann Hospital ultimately would affect that institution and the nature of its eye clinic. In 1941, the Texas legislature took the first steps that ultimately led to the development of the Texas Medical Center by appropriating $500,000 to The University of Texas for the establishment of a cancer research hospital. The M. D. Anderson Foundation offered to match the appropriation if the state would locate the new cancer center in Houston and name it in honor of M. D. Anderson. The Anderson Foundation also helped in attracting the Baylor University School of Medicine to Houston. In February 1946, the M. D. Anderson Foundation presented the deed for 134 acres of land adjacent to Hermann Hospital and Hermann Park to Dr. E. W. Bertner, president of the Texas Medical Center. The land and the opportunity to locate in the new medical facility quickly brought construction of the Baylor medical school, new hospital construction, a library, and a host of other related services.

Hermann Hospital no longer stood alone in the "country," but was now in the midst of a burgeoning, modern medical center. Demand for services grew, to a point where hospital officials eventually broke ground on June 16, 1947 for a new, four hundred–bed addition to Hermann Hospital. The cornerstone was laid in 1948, and the building was completed in February 1949 at a cost of $7.3 million. This was the first addition to the hospital facilities since the original hospital's completion in 1925. By 1954, the completion of Hermann Hospital's "New Building," along with the Hermann Professional Building, Methodist Hospital, the Arabia Temple Crippled Children's Hospital, M. D. Anderson Cancer Hospital, Texas Children's Hospital, St. Luke's Episcopal Hospital, the Jessie Jones Library Building, and the nearly completed new home for the University of Texas Dental Branch added significantly to the overall size of the Texas Medical Center.[17]

But even with all the new construction and the new addition to the hospital, change came slowly to the Hermann Hospital eye clinic. Dr. George R. Kolodny, who came to Houston in 1950 to begin his ophthalmology practice, described the eye clinic at Hermann Hospital as "depressing." He recalled that the clinic occupied two small rooms on the main floor of the old building. "You had to go through a hallway to get to those two little rooms," he stated. "There were no windows; you couldn't see out. The rooms were very tiny. Just big enough to have a place for patients to sit and for you to sit and that was it. It wasn't much of a place."[18]

Dr. Louis Girard, who became chair of the department of ophthalmology at Baylor in 1956, also remembered that there was little in the way of professional training available for ophthalmologists in Houston until the 1950s. As Girard recalled, "In the early 1950s, remember, there was no eye department at Baylor. The eye department was not really started until I came down from New York. Before I came, Dr. Goar... would just go and give lectures to the medical students. There were no residents. And I was the one who started to establish eye departments in the various hospitals." Girard helped to establish the eye service at Ben Taub, the Veteran's Hospital, Methodist Hospital, and at Texas Children's. "And I brought these all under the aegis of the department of ophthalmology at Baylor College of Medicine. So, my residents had an opportunity to rotate through these various hospitals for their training." Girard said that he tried to connect the eye departments at the various hospitals but that he never succeeded in getting Hermann Hospital to be part of that program. "Hermann had their own program and they were not anxious to become part of the Baylor program," said Girard. "I don't think they really got started in expansion and developed their own eye program until Dr. Ruiz started there."[19]

Although the exact date is unclear, evidence suggests that Hermann Hospital launched a modest and somewhat rudimentary ophthalmology residency program during the late 1940s, but possibly as early as 1945. Dr. Elizabeth Crawford recalled:

> There wasn't any program to it. They just hired a resident
> and he worked in the clinic. He would be there every day and
> would do all the refractions and the routine work which the
> staff had had to do before and when you went to the clinic,
> he would have the patients that he wanted you to discuss or
> see there and ready for you to see them. But with just one
> resident, it was more or less of a one-to-one teaching and
> you were talking about the patient that was there. There was
> no such thing as say, "well, we're going to talk about retinas

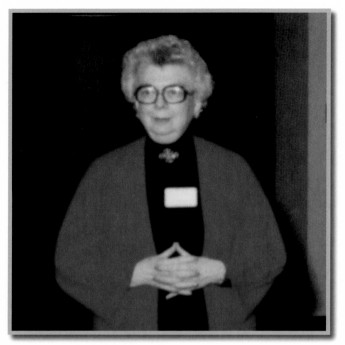

Elizabeth Crawford, MD, circa 1968.

today..." They only had one resident there until the 1950s. They began to get a few pieces of equipment for the clinic and I'd say it was then the first equipment for retinal detachment [photocoagulator] became available in Germany. And I believe that was about 1955, and that was before Dr. [Alice] McPherson and Dr. Ruiz came to Houston as well-trained people in retina problems. [20]

Interestingly, Dick Ruiz recalled that Hermann Hospital's Zeiss Photocoagulator was still in the packing crate when he returned to Hermann Hospital in 1962, primarily because no one there knew how to use it.

George Kolodny credits Tom Royce with taking the initiative to improve the eye clinic and residency training program at Hermann. "As I recall, it was Royce who first insisted on enlarging or getting more space to try to make something more out of it," said Kolodny. "It became a good eye service with Tom Royce. He was interested and wanted it to develop . . . held staff meetings, clinic meetings."[21]

It was this setting that Dr. Richard Ruiz ventured into on July 1, 1957 to begin his medical internship and his introduction to Hermann Hospital. He had not yet chosen a subspecialty, and the hospital's eye service clearly left him unimpressed. But, the field of ophthalmology had become more sophisticated and professional since the days of the early "oculists" in Houston. World-renowned ophthalmologists had developed new surgical techniques, and a new era of research and technological development was about to dawn. As is often the case, fate soon intervened, sending Ruiz on a path that ultimately led him to create an eye center that would emerge from the humble and somewhat shaky origins of the Hermann Hospital eye clinic to become one of the leading eye centers in the nation.

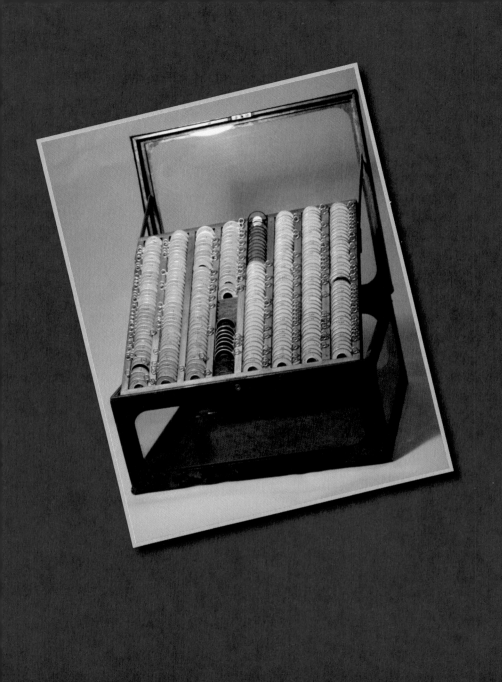

CHAPTER TWO

The Preparation

"I NEVER THOUGHT about being anything but a doctor," said Dick Ruiz. "It never entered my mind to do anything else." Ruiz acknowledged that his father, Dr. John J. Ruiz Sr., was a major influence in his career choice. "It was not that he would sit me down and tell me how wonderful it was to be a physician, but I just watched him and I saw the respect that he garnered by being a physician, and the affection a lot of his patients had for him." Over the years, Ruiz saw his father help many people, some of whom simply lacked the financial means to pay for their treatment. All of this had a profound impact on a young man growing up in 1940s Houston.[1]

Richard S. Ruiz came from a long line of hard-working, entrepreneurial people. His paternal grandfather, Quentin Ruiz, migrated to Mexico from the little town of Puente Arce, near Santander, in northern Spain. In time, he met Maria Fernandez, an Italian Mexican from Brownsville, Texas. The couple married and settled in Huatusco, a coffee growing area about fifty miles inland from Veracruz, where Quentin Ruiz made a good living in the coffee processing and distribution business. Here, they raised thirteen children: ten boys and three girls. They believed strongly in the benefits of a good education and sent all of the boys to St. Mary's Catholic School, a private school in Kentucky. While all of his brothers eventually returned to Mexico, Richard Ruiz's father,

Juan José (John Joseph), one of the younger children of the family, stayed in the United States, where he attended The University of Texas School of Pharmacy, which was located in Galveston at that time. Graduating in 1925, he was in one of the last classes before the university moved its pharmacy school to Austin during the summer of 1927.[2]

While attending pharmacy school in Galveston, Ruiz met his future bride, a woman of Irish Mexican antecedents named Luz Stranahan. Her father was an Irish American road and bridge engineer from Huntsville, Texas. While doing some work for the Mexican government, Stranahan met his future wife, Maria. The couple eventually married and settled on a ranch near Mazatlán in the western Mexican state of Sinaloa. Here, Luz was born the third of seven children, a few years before the outbreak of the Mexican Revolution that began in November 1910. As the situation worsened, most Americans in the area, including the Stranahan family, were evacuated by battleship to San Diego, California. Eventually, Stranahan brought his wife and young family to Texas. Two years after they arrived in Galveston, Stranahan died of pneumonia, leaving a wife who spoke only Spanish and six surviving children, all under the age of seventeen. Stranahan's sudden death left his family in dire economic circumstances, and all of the children, including fourteen-year-old Luz, pitched in to help. In time, all of the girls worked either for the Moody National Bank or the American National Insurance Company (ANICO). The eldest son, George, ultimately landed an office job with the Santa Fe Railroad.

Sometime during these years, 1921–25, Luz Stranahan and John J. Ruiz met and subsequently married. Following his graduation from The University of Texas School of Pharmacy in 1925, the couple moved to Houston where John Ruiz took a job at a Fannin Street pharmacy called Prescription House. Later, he opened his own drugstore on Canal Street near McAlpine. During the next seven years, Ruiz ran his *farmacia*, and the couple's family began with the arrival of John Joseph Jr. Eighteen months later, on July 12, 1932, a second son, Ricardo (Richard) Strana-

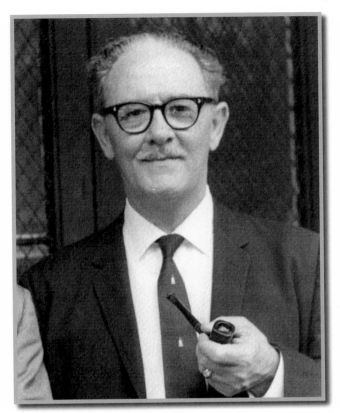

John J. Ruiz, MD, circa 1960.

han Ruiz arrived. John Ruiz had begun taking pre-med courses at Houston Junior College (now the University of Houston), and in 1932, about six weeks after the arrival of his second child, he entered medical school at The University of Texas Medical Branch in Galveston. While he was a medical student, the family increased in size with the arrival of a third child, Dolores.[3]

Although he had wanted to become a pediatrician, these were the years of the Great Depression and John Ruiz simply did not have the luxury of taking the extra time needed to train in pediatrics while simultaneously supporting his young and growing family. Following graduation from UTMB in 1936, he interned at Methodist Hospital on San Jacinto Street in downtown Houston. After the completion of his internship, he went into family

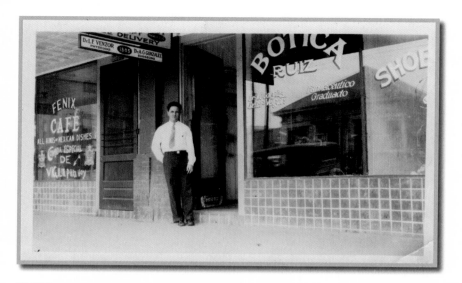

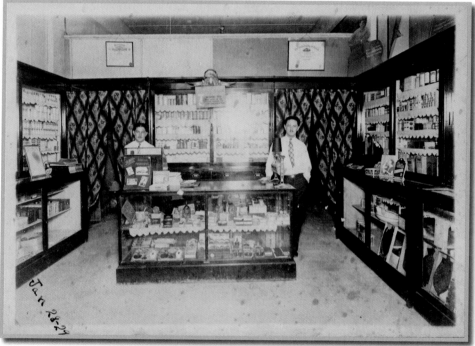

Top, Dr. John Ruiz in front of his pharmacy. Bottom, Interior of Botica Ruiz, 1929.

practice. Ruiz decided to build his medical practice in the same neighborhood where his pharmacy had been. The following year he opened an office on Navigation, in a small three-room space situated in the Crespo Funeral Home building, across from Our Lady of Guadalupe Church. In 1944, he moved to Park Place, near Houston Municipal Airport (now William P. Hobby Airport). Dr. John Ruiz's practice grew rapidly, and during World War II he was exceedingly busy, in part because so many younger medical doctors had been called to active duty in the armed forces.

Childhood was a happy time for Dick Ruiz. "We lived well," he recalled. "Not ostentatiously at all, but we always had enough to eat and a roof over our heads. My mom was a great cook—she learned from her mother and was just one of those special cooks." Ruiz recalled that his father had few hobbies, but enjoyed playing tennis and occasional poker games with some of his friends. He remembered his father mainly as a serious man who focused on his medical practice. But, concerning his children, "My dad was just a fanatic about education and he believed that the key to a successful life was to be trained in a profession." Ruiz acknowledged that his father was a major influence throughout his life and definitely in his decision to pursue a career in medicine. "But I do not remember him urging me to be a physician. He was a firm believer in education, and though he thought the medical profession was best of all, I am sure that had I decided to pursue another profession, he would have been very supportive. He would tell me, 'Just get the education and get as much as you can.'"

Most of John Ruiz's brothers and sisters settled in northern Mexico, primarily around Torreón and Monterrey. Although the Ruiz family did not travel very often, they did enjoy periodic visits with John Ruiz's family in Mexico. "Once in a while, Dad wanted to go see his mother and his family, and that was always fun. My uncle Raymond had a ranch near Cadereyta Jiménez, about fifty miles north of Monterrey. We spent probably two, maybe three summers up there on his ranch and got to ride a lot of horses when we were young."[4]

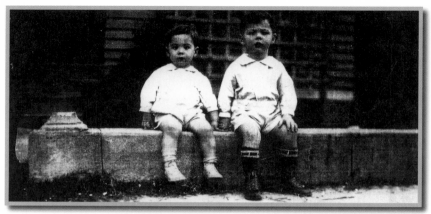

Brothers—Dick and Johnny Ruiz, circa 1935.

Dick Ruiz loved riding horses during his childhood years. Knowing this, one of Dr. John's friends boarded a horse with the Ruiz family. In return for caring for the horse, a beautiful palomino named Penney, the Ruiz children could ride whenever they wished. "We lived right on the edge of the city limit at that time, right up against Sims Bayou," said Ruiz. "Our lot extended down to the bayou, about three quarters of an acre. We had an old garage with three stalls in it and we made one of them into a horse stall." Several families in the area kept horses, and the young people in the neighborhood often rode together. "We used to have a lot of fun on that horse, but he was a lot of trouble to take care of." One of Ruiz's riding companions introduced him to her friend, Yvonne Mosher. "Yvonne went to Incarnate Word Academy," said Ruiz. "She was raised on the east side, too. We met during the summer before high school, and we started going together very shortly thereafter. It was kind of love at first sight!"

Dick Ruiz also attended Catholic schools including Blessed Sacrament, St. Christopher's, and then St. Thomas High School, on the corner of Memorial Drive and Shepherd in Houston. It was a long way to the campus for the Ruiz boys, nearly two hours of combined walking and riding city buses. After a year or so of this, young John Ruiz got his first car, a 1936 Ford. There were no freeways in those days and part of the one-hour drive was down a stretch of humpbacked, two-lane road. Despite the long commute, Dick Ruiz found time to participate in school activities and for four years lettered in basketball. "I made a lot of good friends there that are still good friends," he recalled. "It was a great school. Still is a great school. I have nothing but fond memories of it—the good old days!"

Even as a young man, Dick Ruiz was a very determined individual. Upon graduation from St. Thomas High School in 1951, he enrolled at Texas A&M and began attending summer classes. After two intense years of classes at A&M, with supplementary courses at the University of Houston and Arlington State, Ruiz was accepted into medical school at UTMB in Galveston. And finally, after an eight-year courtship that lasted through high school and into medical school, Dick and Yvonne married on June 11, 1955, following his sophomore year at UTMB.

Although Dick Ruiz was resolute in his determination to become a physician, early on he was not so sure about which area of specialization to pursue. Initially, he had been interested in psychiatry, but later changed his mind and decided to focus on internal medicine. "By the time I finished medical school," Ruiz later recalled, "I was going to go into internal medicine because I was very influenced by the professor of medicine, Raymond Gregory, who was a great physician, a great teacher, and just a terrific diagnostician." As part of the senior year in medical school, students were required to participate in a three-month preceptorship. This was a means of introducing senior medical students to family practice and also to the rural communities of Texas, which needed more medical doctors. The school had made arrangements with a number of family practice physicians to host students and provide them with guided experience in their offices. Although the students generally had to go to a rural community, the school made an exception for Dick Ruiz since he had a wife and their first child at home. He did his preceptorship "on the other side of town," in the office of Dr. Mylie Durham Jr., in the Heights.

Durham's father, Dr. Mylie Durham Sr., was one of the founders of the Heights Hospital. Durham Sr. had two sons, both of whom had become doctors. Mylie Durham Jr. was in family practice, and his younger brother, Charles, specialized in obstetrics and gynecology. At the time, Durham Sr. still was seeing some patients in family practice. Another family practitioner, Nick Adamo, and an internist, Guy Purnell, were also part of the clinic. During this preceptorship, Ruiz saw firsthand what the private practice of internal medicine outside of an academic institution entailed. As he described it later, Ruiz said, "I had the opportunity to see the private practice of internal medicine—vis-à-vis the practice of the professor of medicine at Galveston, who was seeing these fascinating cases and diagnostic dilemmas—and I changed my mind." Dr. Gregory generally saw many challenging cases that were referred to him from across the state. But in private practice, "it was colds, sniffles, and an occasional ulcer," said Ruiz. "And I did not want to do that." He wanted to specialize in an area that would challenge him and enable him to make a real difference in the lives of his patients.[5]

With this experience in mind, Ruiz was uncertain about what area of medicine to pursue. His father suggested that he consider a residency in general medicine, an additional year of general surgery, and then join him in his family practice. But Dick Ruiz saw that the trend in medicine was toward more specialization. In July 1957, the newly graduated Dr. Richard S. Ruiz started a rotating internship at Hermann Hospital. Here the interns rotated through different services including urology, anesthesia, orthopedics, general medicine, and surgery. They also had a mandatory, one-month emergency room rotation with twelve-hour shifts. "I started in the emergency room," said Ruiz, "at night, right out of medical school!" In the emergency room, the interns felt the pressure of being the "only doctor" on duty, although medical residents were nearby and always on call if needed. "But they did not like to be bothered unless it was really necessary, so you really felt that responsibility of being a green, young guy right out of medical school." Interestingly, the eye service was not one of the major programs in Hermann Hospital at that time. Thinking back, Ruiz noted, "I remember when I was an intern in 1957–58; there was one eye resident in this hospital, a fellow from Brazil named Paolo Baras. The eye clinic was on the east end of the ground floor of the original building. The clinic itself was one big room about twenty by thirty feet. There was a little vestibule-like area and then a small waiting room, and that was the eye clinic."[6]

Ruiz found that he enjoyed surgery and decided he would choose a surgical specialty. He talked with several doctors, including friends of his father and many others, seeking their advice and opinions. Most of them had become intrigued with the field of ophthalmology as an area that held great promise for the future. During his internship at Hermann Hospital, Dick Ruiz met another medical intern, Whitney Sampson, and the two hit it off as friends. Sampson, a graduate of Baylor College of Medicine, had decided early to go into ophthalmology. His enthusiasm for ophthalmology impressed Ruiz, who began to think seriously about that field of medicine. Coincidentally, around this time, due in part to a family emergency, Ruiz was involved in an event that proved to be "the moment" when he knew in his heart that ophthalmology was the career for which he was destined.

Ruiz's aunt Helen, his mother's sister, developed a case of acute glaucoma. She had been referred to Dr. Ralph Dunn, an ophthalmologist, who had an office in the Hermann Professional Building. Ruiz's aunt was admitted to Hermann Hospital by Dunn for further treatment. When she did not respond satisfactorily to treatment, he determined that she needed emergency surgery. Knowing that Ruiz was contemplating the field of ophthalmology, Dunn invited him to scrub with him and assist in the procedure. "So, at 10 o'clock at night, we took her down to surgery and, of course, she was my aunt, so I was involved from that standpoint," said Ruiz. "At that time, I was getting interested in ophthalmology and I went to scrub with him on this emergency cataract operation to relieve the acute glaucoma. And, that sort of did it, you know—it hooked me." After the surgery, Ruiz was excited about what he witnessed in the operating room and discussed ophthalmology and training with Dunn. Dunn had studied at the Kresge Eye Institute at Wayne State University in Detroit. "He felt that it was very good training and a good place. He seemed to be a pretty sharp ophthalmologist. And so, that is how I got into ophthalmology."[7]

Convinced from his discussion with Dunn that Wayne State University and its Kresge Eye Institute in Detroit was the place he wanted to study, Ruiz applied for a residency. But time was passing and it was getting late in the process for him to apply for admission as a resident. Ruiz called the office of the chair of ophthalmology, Dr. A. D. Ruedemann, to request an application packet. He promptly completed it and waited for a reply. "I never heard a thing," Ruiz recalled. "One month went by... Two months went by... Three months went by... Now, it was getting into the spring, you know, and a new group started in July. So, I was putting all my eggs in one basket, and I was not hearing anything." Ruiz took the initiative and called to request a meeting with Dr. Ruedemann. The secretary set an appointment for a meeting in the city/county hospital eye clinic at 9:00 AM on the next Sunday. The hospital was the main level-1 trauma center and emergency room for the greater Detroit area, and therefore, had a very busy emergency room. Ruiz arrived in Detroit on Friday afternoon. Early on Saturday morning he met the resident on call, Dr. Edward Isby. "I just hung around with him all day long," said Ruiz. "I wanted to see what it was like there, and I was very impressed. Isby was passionate about ophthalmology and he also loved to teach, so that really solidified my interest." Ruiz stayed with Isby until late in the evening and then returned to his hotel, several blocks away.

Early the next morning, Ruiz returned to the hospital eagerly, if nervously, anticipating his meeting with Dr. Ruedemann. "I must have gotten to the hospital one hour early, and I went into the eye clinic. Of course, there was no clinic on Sunday so it was just like a tomb in there. They had metal benches in the waiting area, two-and-a-half feet apart, long benches where you could seat about ten to fifteen people, a typical charity clinic–type deal. And so I sat in there." Time passed, and still there was no sign of Dr. Ruedemann. Shortly after 10:00 AM, two residents walked through and saw Ruiz, dressed in a suit and tie, and obviously waiting for someone. The residents called Dr. Ruedemann, who had returned after making his rounds at Harper Hospital. Ruedemann spoke to Ruiz and assured him that he would drive immediately to meet him at the receiving clinic.

Before coming to Wayne State, Dr. Ruedemann had served as head of ophthalmology at the Cleveland Clinic. He was known to be a hard-working, independent thinker with a fiery personality and was described as being outspoken and frequently "colorful" in his speech. In Cleveland, he developed a large following and generally saw "an extraordinarily large number of patients on a daily basis." After years of confrontation with the clinic's chief of surgery, Dr. Thomas E. Jones, the fiercely independent Ruedemann left the Cleveland Clinic in 1947 to take the position as chair and professor of ophthalmology at Wayne State. The following year, Dr. Ruedemann and Dr. Parker Heath, the former chair of ophthalmology, secured a grant from the Kresge Foundation and established the Kresge Eye Institute, with the goal of bringing together physicians and scientists in a collaborative setting to develop better techniques for preserving vision.[8]

Fifty years after their first meeting, Ruiz recalled Dr. Ruedemann as being an affable, warm person. The two sat on a metal bench in the clinic for the interview. "We just started chatting," Ruiz recalled. "He did not ask me any real pointed questions about why I was going into ophthalmology. I told him a little bit about my background: that my dad was a doctor and so on. I remembered that the residents had advised me how important it was to convince Dr. Ruedemann that I really wanted to be an ophthalmologist and that I really wanted to do my residency at Wayne State. He never made any commitment, of course, but he was, I thought, sort of positively responding." After the brief interview, Ruedemann dropped Ruiz off at his hotel. "You will be hearing from us," Ruiz recalls him saying. "He thanked me for coming and that was it."[9]

Ruiz returned to Houston to wait for word from Wayne State. Once again, the exasperating process dragged on. Finally, he called Dr. Ruedemann's office, only to be told that they would contact him soon. Realizing that time was getting short if he were to begin a residency in the coming cycle—it was already May—Dick Ruiz decided that he should also apply to Baylor College of Medicine in Houston. Finally, several days later, he received the news that he had been waiting to hear: Wayne State accepted him into their ophthalmology program. At about the same time, Ruiz also learned that he had been accepted into the ophthalmology program at Baylor, where Dr. Louis Girard was department chairman. His goal always had been to attend Wayne State, and his good friend Whitney Sampson also had enrolled, so without hesitation, Ruiz accepted the residency at Wayne State.[10]

Ruiz, who by now was the father of two young daughters, temporarily left his wife and family in Houston and traveled to Detroit. He had to find housing for his family and then report to Wayne State to begin his residency. Ruiz stayed at the home of Ed and Roxanne Isby, who graciously hosted him for a full two weeks until he found a suitable place and could make arrangements to move his family to Detroit. With the help of the eye clinic's secretary, he found a small, furnished, brick house with a fenced back yard located conveniently near a bus line. This was of great benefit since Ruiz did not have a car. After one year, the landlady was so taken with the young family that she reduced the rent from $125 to $110 a month, allowing them to stay for the full three years of Ruiz's residency.[11]

While they were in Detroit, Yvonne became pregnant with their third child. Unknown to Dick and Yvonne, a fourth child was on the way too. "And the interesting thing about it is, they [twins] were completely undiagnosed," said Dick Ruiz. "So, we had two girls already, and in those days, you did not know whether it was going to be a boy or girl." As was the practice at the time, Ruiz remained in the waiting room with the other nervous fathers while his wife was taken to the delivery room. Having already had two children, he knew what to expect. When the delivery took longer than anticipated, however, Ruiz became worried. Finally, the doctor emerged and said, "Dick, sit down. You just had twin boys." The doctor announced that mother and children were doing fine. Ruiz, who had been hoping for a son, recalled later, "That was a terrific surprise!" He realized that he had much to do before his wife and the new babies came home. Ruiz had been moonlighting at night in local emergency rooms to make extra money: $35 a night for a twelve-hour shift. He had arranged to borrow a bassinette for the new baby from one of the small hospitals where he was working, but now had to hustle to get more supplies. "I thought there was going to be one baby, so I had to do some real scampering around, get another bassinette and more diapers— there were no disposable diapers then. But it was a lot of fun." With four small children, the Ruiz household was always abuzz with activity and energy. "You know, I never remember Yvonne complaining about all of the work. Not one time. It just amazes me. She could not even go to the drug store or the grocery store. You have four little kids like that, you just cannot manage them. So, we got this twin stroller, but you could not even go on the sidewalk because nobody could stay on the walk with you."[12]

During their three years in Detroit, Yvonne took care of the young Ruiz kids while Dick primarily focused on his training and studies. Ruiz described the program as a "combination of residency programs" that included the Wayne State program, which was centered on the Detroit Receiving Hospital and the Kresge Eye Institute. Residents from Harper Hospital and Mount Sinai Hospital rotated through the Receiving Hospital to gain emergency room and clinic experience. This enabled them to treat patients with a variety of illnesses and injuries that one normally did not encounter in the typical private practice.[13]

Formal teaching lectures were not a major component of the program, with the exception of a basic science course, offered by the Kresge Eye Institute, that all first-year residents in the greater Detroit area attended. The basic science course in ophthalmol-

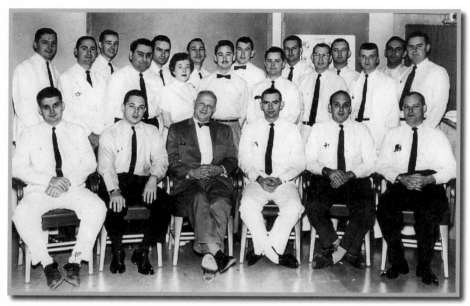

Front row wearing suit, A.D. Ruedemann, MD, with ophthalmology residents, Kresge Eye Institute, Wayne State University, 1959. Dick Ruiz is behind Ruedemann.

ogy consisted of daily, half-day, didactic (formal lecture) sessions for nine months during the first year of training. Ruiz and the six other residents in his group—Ralph Anderson, Craig George, Frank Moran, Patricia Murphy, James Rupple, and William Slack—formed their own journal club, developing a competition to see who would be first to have read and be able to cite the most articles. Ed Isby, a senior resident, joined in to provide additional academic stimulus. The residents were on their own most of the time and were not as closely supervised as they would be in most teaching hospitals today. Wayne State provided some of the best training in the country at that time, and residents generally left with high regard for the program and for Dr. Ruedemann. "He was a real character," Ruiz recalled fondly, "a big bull of a guy with a warm, outgoing personality. He was a real kind-hearted man who cared for his residents—all the residents loved him."[14]

Ruiz completed his residency at Wayne State and Kresge Eye Institute in June 1961. "When I finished there, I thought I had seen just about every thing there was to see in ophthalmology, and that I had done about everything there was to do—including a lot of surgery—and I felt pretty confident." With a wife and four young children to support, he was ready to go to work. His father had been helping with expenses, and Dick felt it was now time to take full responsibility for his family. His father, however, had a good, intuitive sense about medicine and the value of additional training. He advised his son to take yet another year of additional study. "I always listened to him," said Ruiz. "So then, the question in my mind was what to do with an additional year? Take it in what subspecialty?" Ruiz saw two significant opportunities: he could go to New York and study corneal surgery under Dr. Ramon Castroviejo, or pursue a second option: to study under Dr. Charles Schepens, an expert in retinal surgery at the Massachusetts Eye and Ear Infirmary of the Harvard Medical School in Boston. Both men were internationally renowned for groundbreaking work in their subspecialties. A fellowship with either would provide Ruiz with the opportunity to improve his own expertise, enhancing his credentials significantly.

Ramon Castroviejo, the son of an ophthalmologist, was born in Logroño, Spain, in 1904. He graduated from the University of Madrid in 1927 with a degree in medicine. Castroviejo came to the United States in 1928, serving first as an attending ophthalmologist at the Chicago Eye, Ear, Nose, and Throat Hospital. In 1931, after completing a research fellowship at the Mayo Clinic, he went to the Columbia Presbyterian Medical Center in New York, where he later performed the first successful human cornea transplant. Dr. Castroviejo was known internationally for his pioneering surgical and corneal tissue transplant techniques and for designing many innovative ophthalmic instruments.[15]

Charles L. Schepens was born in Mouscron, Belgium, March 13, 1912. Although his father was a physician, Schepens initially studied mathematics before turning to medicine at the State University of Ghent. After graduating from medical school in 1935, he studied ophthalmology at Moorfields Eye Hospital in London.[16] During World War II, he served as a medical officer in the Belgian Air Force until German troops overran the country. Following the German victory, he escaped to France, where he served in the French Resistance under the alias Jacques Perot, a lumber mill operator. He was captured twice by the Gestapo, but managed to escape both times. Finally, he fled to England after learning that the Germans had caught on to his secret operation. In 1947, Schepens came to the United States and became a fellow at the Howe Laboratory of Ophthalmology at the Massachusetts Eye and Ear Infirmary, a primary teaching hospital of the Harvard Medical School. Here he developed the retinal service in ophthalmology. In 1949, Schepens established the first retina service and the first retinal disease fellowship at the Massachusetts Eye and Ear Infirmary. The following year, he founded the Retina Foundation to conduct research in retinal disease (now known as the Schepens Eye Research Institute, affiliated with Harvard Medical School). Among his professional accomplishments, Schepens invented the binocular indirect ophthalmoscope (BIO), an instrument that enabled ophthalmologists to see the entire retina in three dimensions. He built the original prototype from scraps of metal he recovered from the streets of London during the Blitz. He led the way in innovative surgical techniques, including scleral buckling to repair retinal detachments. His techniques improved the success rate in retinal surgery from about 40 percent to 80 percent. Schepens trained over 170 vitreoretinal surgeons, wrote four books, and published over 340 research papers during his long career. Schepens and his associates combined clinical practice with eye research and teaching. More than anyone else, he raised the standard of care for the treatment of retinal disease throughout the world.[17]

Ruiz, with two excellent opportunities from which to choose, traveled to New York to meet Dr. Castroviejo and discuss a possible fellowship. "He was one of the real pioneers in corneal transplantation—a marvelous surgeon," said Ruiz. "He published extensively on cataract surgery and corneal transplantation." Ruiz had met Dr. Schepens and some of his associates previously at an American Academy of Ophthalmology meeting in Chicago. "The thing that I felt the least competent in was retina," Ruiz later re-called. At the time, retina research and treatment was emerging as a promising subspecialty. Although Dr. Castroviejo had offered him a fellowship in New York, Ruiz was greatly intrigued with the retina program at the Massachusetts Eye and Ear Infirmary/Harvard Medical School. "I was very impressed with how organized the program was. I could see that it was going to be a much more didactic, more organized, more predictable type of training program and Massachusetts Eye and Ear Infirmary had one of the best reputations in the world for training in ophthalmology. So, I decided to go that route."

Ruiz accepted the fellowship offer from Dr. Schepens and

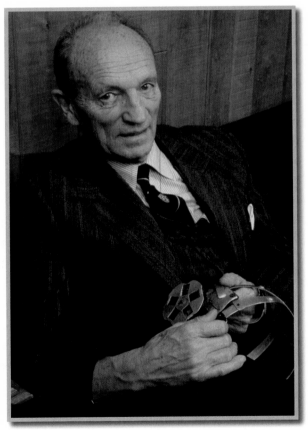

Charles Schepens, MD, with prototype of his Indirect Ophthalmoscope.

moved his family from Detroit to Boston. This decision proved to be one of the most important in Ruiz's career, because he would spend the next year studying under a man widely known as a pioneer in modern retinal surgery. The significance of this opportunity was not lost on Ruiz. "Schepens was already very well known and the group that was around him was well known. They published a lot and they were right at the forefront of retinal surgery in the world. There is no question about it. It was the place in the world to get retinal training—Massachusetts Eye and Ear Infirmary, affiliated with Harvard Medical School, and the second-oldest eye hospital (founded in 1824) in the United States." The Howe Laboratory of Ophthalmology at Harvard Medical School was on the cutting edge of research, providing the opportunity for Ruiz to explore the latest in diagnoses and treatments. He further developed his surgical skills and became comfortable using the indirect ophthalmoscope, gaining a high level of expertise in one of the most difficult subspecialties in ophthalmology. "It was more one-on-one training and when you first got there," said Ruiz years later, "the biggest challenge was learning to use the instrument [indirect ophthalmoscope]. It literally takes about one hundred hours of practice to learn to use the instrument properly and after that, you can begin to learn to interpret. It was a very, very difficult process to go through ... because the technique was so difficult." Ruiz recalled that the clinical care of patients "was clearly a higher level of care than existed in the country at that time in general." He found the academic part of the program challenging and stimulating: "a different dimension" adding to a regimen that essentially immersed the fellows in all of the latest scientific, diagnostic, and technological developments related to the retina.[18]

As Ruiz's fellowship with Dr. Schepens drew to a close in 1962, he began to explore opportunities to open an ophthalmology practice in Houston. Dr. Schepens asked Ruiz to stay for another year, and he had received several offers in Detroit, but Ruiz knew in his heart that he wanted to come back home to Houston and practice at Hermann Hospital. He contacted Dr. Thomas

Royce, chief of ophthalmology at the hospital, and learned that Royce, along with Drs. Elizabeth Crawford, George Kolodny, Marion Johnson, and several other ophthalmologists were forming a group practice. After completing his fellowship in retina with Dr. Schepens, Ruiz would bring a special expertise to any group practice. Royce invited Ruiz to meet with him to discuss joining the group. But after flying from Boston for the meeting, Ruiz was disappointed at the offer and also at what seemed like uncertainty regarding how the practice would be organized. The salary was less than he anticipated and the lack of focus in how the practice would operate gnawed at him, too. Ruiz conferred with his father and decided not to accept the offer.[19]

But this meant that the future still was uncertain, and Ruiz had to make some decisions quickly. His fellowship was about to end, he had a family to support, and he was anxious to begin his professional practice. Ruiz knew that he wanted to establish his practice in Houston and that he wanted to work at Hermann Hospital and in the Texas Medical Center. He had fond memories of his internship at Hermann; he had made many friends, including Dr. Leigh Crozier, CEO of the hospital. "I always wanted to come back to Hermann Hospital," said Ruiz. "I wanted to do all my work here because I really loved this hospital." Crozier was a pioneer in hospital administration and had been very supportive of Ruiz. "He liked me because I was interested in the teaching program, and I was also interested in the hospital."[20]

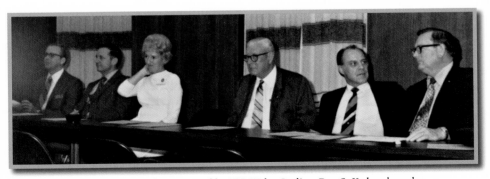

From left, Unknown, Neill Amsler, Betty Hadden RN, Walter Sterling, Dan G. Kadvrach, and Dixon Manley, Hermann Hospital/Hermann Hospital Estate, circa 1965.

Although he did not realize it at the time, Dick Ruiz was about to make a decision that would affect not only his family, but in time, thousands of people who one day would become patients of the Hermann Eye Center. Deciding to open his own practice, he contacted Dixon Manley and Neill F. Amsler Jr., administrators of the Hermann Hospital Estate, which managed both Hermann Hospital and the Hermann Professional Building. He explained his desire to open an office in the Hermann Professional Building and to practice at Hermann Hospital. It turned out that Dr. Elizabeth Crawford, a well respected Houston ophthalmologist, was vacating her office on the eleventh floor of the Hermann Professional Building to join the new group practice. The location, about 1,500 square feet in size, was ideal, but the monthly rent seemed rather pricey ($1.00 per square foot) for a young doctor who was just beginning his medical practice. He returned to Boston to consider the offer and other options that might be available. Not one to give up on an idea, Ruiz again contacted Dixon Manley to discuss the rental terms. Manley, perhaps at the suggestion of Dr. Crozier and with the stipulation that no major remodeling would be done, offered the space to Ruiz at a 50 percent discount for the first year to help launch his practice. Now that he had secured office space, a very happy Dick Ruiz began making arrangements, by long distance no less, to acquire enough furnishings and equipment to open his practice. Ruiz completed his fellowship in Boston at the end of June, packed his family into their car and set out for Houston. "I had a little Rambler station wagon," he remembered later. With the four kids and no air conditioning, the drive to Houston "was pretty darned hot."

On July 9, 1962, Dr. Richard S. Ruiz opened his ophthalmology practice on the eleventh floor of the Hermann Professional Building, directly across the street from Hermann Hospital. His lifelong dream of practicing medicine in his hometown was about to become a reality. The years of intense preparation lay behind, and ahead would be the task of building an ophthalmology practice. He had studied under some of the leading ophthalmologists

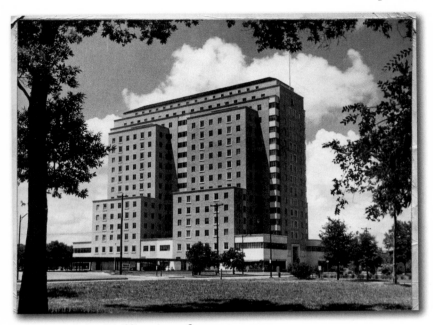

Hermann Professional Building, circa 1962.

in the world and would build upon that knowledge in developing his own expertise. Research in ophthalmology was showing great potential for new understanding and treatment of vision problems. Scientists and engineers were developing new miniaturized technology that would enable surgeons to perform almost miraculous feats in repairing sick and damaged eyes. Richard Ruiz was beginning his career in ophthalmology during one of the most extraordinary periods in the history of medicine. He had prepared well and now embraced the opportunities in research and the opportunity to share these exciting developments with new doctors who would be training at Hermann Hospital. There was a lot of hard work ahead, but during the next few years, while he built up a practice and settled in at Hermann Hospital, an idea would begin to crystallize in Ruiz's mind about creating a world-class eye center. What began as a solo ophthalmology practice on a steamy July morning in 1962 would in a few years develop into one of the premier eye centers in the country, and it would do so in the heart of Houston's own Texas Medical Center.

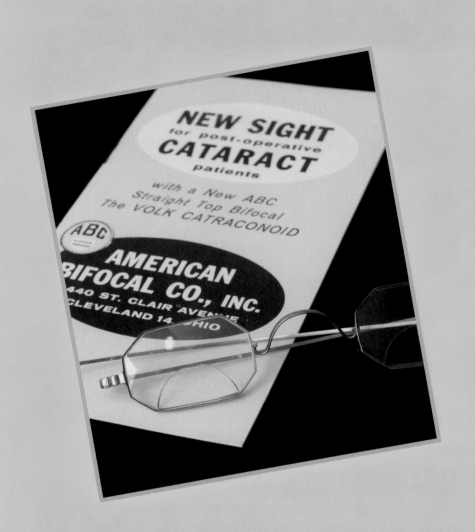

CHAPTER THREE

Building a Practice

"I" WANTED TO DO MY WORK at Hermann, I wanted to put my office in the Hermann Professional Building, and I wanted to be involved in the training program." On July 9, 1962, Dr. Richard S. Ruiz formally opened his ophthalmology practice in an eleventh floor office of the Hermann Professional Building. The building stood in a prominent location, across from Hermann Hospital on Fannin Street, at the northern end of the booming Texas Medical Center. Before he opened his office, Ruiz had faced a monumental decision: whether to limit his practice to his subspecialty—retina—or begin a general ophthalmology practice with an emphasis on retina. This decision was crucial because it would determine the scope of his medical practice and teaching for the rest of his career. Although a practice limited to retina would have been very lucrative, Ruiz instead chose the general ophthalmology path. He believed that one of the most rewarding aspects of general ophthalmology was the opportunity to see the same patients year after year, forging lifelong bonds with them and gaining their trust. He liked the idea of getting to know his patients and providing eye care for them and later, for their children and even their grandchildren. In a general ophthalmology practice, Ruiz could do the kind of traditional doctoring—broadly defined—that would be similar to his father's experience in family practice. He looked forward

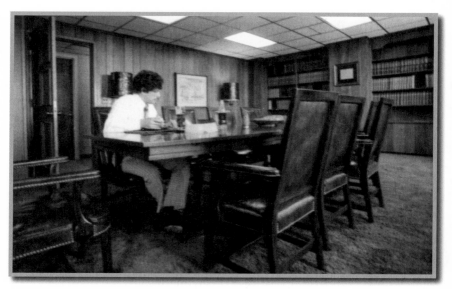

Houston Eye Associates Conference Room—Hermann Professional Building.

not only to his role as a physician, but also to the social interaction and to being a trusted confidante for his patients. By having a general ophthalmology practice, Ruiz could have the best of both worlds: providing lifelong care for many patients and still having ample opportunities to work in his subspecialty. In addition, with a general ophthalmology practice, Ruiz would be less dependent on other doctors for patient referrals. He could cultivate a broad base of patients and also continue to develop his expertise not only in retina, but in general ophthalmology. Dick Ruiz knew that he wanted to be involved in teaching and that a general ophthalmology practice would provide a broad range of clinical experience and enhance his ability as a teacher.

Thus, having made this monumental decision, Ruiz now could begin to fulfill his dream of practicing medicine and teaching in conjunction with the ophthalmology residency program at Hermann Hospital. He would build a very successful ophthalmology practice over the next ten years, create a multi-specialty eye clinic by bringing associates with fellowship training in specific areas of expertise into one office, take a major leadership role as one of the youngest chiefs of a service at Hermann Hospital, direct the eye service at M. D. Anderson Cancer Center, and serve as chief of the eye service at St. Joseph's Hospital.[1]

Building a medical practice from scratch, however, was a daunting challenge that required determination, ambition, and dedication. Ruiz worked many long, hard hours treating patients in a variety of locations and making himself known in the community. He had to overcome several other hurdles as well. His eleventh floor office was not in a location that attracted "walk-in" patients and he faced stiff competition in the same building from many well-established ophthalmologists including, ironically, the new ophthalmology group practice spearheaded by Dr. Thomas Royce.[2] Still, Ruiz showed the tenacity and determination with which he approached every major challenge as he set out to establish his own ophthalmology practice. His first office in the Hermann Professional Building, a space previously occupied by Dr. Elizabeth Crawford, was about 1,500 square feet and included a waiting room, two treatment rooms, a small lab room, and an office-reception area. Reminiscing years later, Ruiz said, "That was not very big, but it sure sounded big to me!" He signed a five-year lease, borrowed $50,000 from his uncle Raymond to buy equipment and furnishings, and opened his office with one staff person, nurse Hazel Haltom. "She was great," he recalled, "and she worked with me for a long time." As he began seeing patients, Ruiz did his best to meet other doctors in the Medical Center, encouraging them to send their eye patients to him. "I was going around shaking hands all over this medical center, telling people I was here and would love to see their patients and . . . getting down to that [Hermann Hospital] doctors' dining room where doctors gathered for coffee and conversation every morning before they made their medical rounds."[3]

Ruiz worked almost anywhere and everywhere that he could to see patients and build his practice. He secured a staff appointment at St. Joseph's Hospital, where his father had practiced for many years, and began doing eye surgery there on Thursdays.

Tuesdays were surgery days at Hermann Hospital, and on Tuesday afternoons and Saturdays he saw patients at his father's Park Place clinic on the east side of Houston. Dr. John Ruiz designed his small clinic so that two doctors could make use of the space. Dick Ruiz remembered that it had a small office in the front that he made into an exam room. His father had one employee, Mrs. Inez Menifee, who had been with him for over twenty years. She was trained as a lab technician and performed all of the other tasks in the office including nursing, X-rays, and taking appointments. "She made my appointments for me and I would go out there every Tuesday afternoon and Saturday afternoon," said Ruiz. "That was a real God-send because my dad ... sent me more patients than anybody. He had patients lined up waiting for me when I came back to Houston." In the struggle to build a practice and pay his bills, Ruiz gratefully recalled, "I made my living on Saturdays for the first two years." Among the other doctors Ruiz approached for patient referrals was Dr. James Hayes, a medical school colleague of his father. The senior Ruiz befriended Hayes years before, and Hayes was delighted to invite Dick Ruiz to open a small eye clinic in his Alvin, Texas, hospital, where he would see eye patients one day a week. The early years then, were very hectic for Ruiz. With office hours in the Hermann Professional Building, surgery at St. Joseph's and Hermann hospitals, and clinic hours in Alvin and at his father's office, Ruiz really had to hustle to keep up with his schedule and build up his medical practice.[4]

While working to establish an ophthalmology practice, Ruiz also pursued his interest in academics. During his years in medical school, he had discovered both a knack for and a love of teaching. After returning to Houston, he quickly secured faculty appointments and did retina consulting at both Baylor College of Medicine and at UTMB in Galveston. Ruiz loved UTMB and made the weekly trek to Galveston every Friday afternoon for fifteen years, until the Hermann Eye Center opened in the Jones Pavilion in 1977. If events had unfolded a little differently, Ruiz might well have ended up permanently in Galveston instead of Houston.

While he was completing his fellowship in Boston with Dr. Schepens, Ruiz had written to Dr. Wendell Gingrich, chair of ophthalmology at UTMB, inquiring if there were any opportunities for him to teach on a part-time basis. Ruiz wanted to secure an academic appointment and also believed that by working with the residents, he would make it more possible for them to get acquainted with him, develop confidence in his abilities, and refer retina patients to him once they began their own practices. Apparently, Gingrich misinterpreted Ruiz's intention and recommended him for a full-time career development award with the Public Health Service. Ruiz replied and politely turned down the full-time opportunity, but stated that he would get in touch with Dr. Gingrich once he returned to Houston. After Ruiz signed a five-year lease and opened his office in the Hermann Professional Building, he contacted Gingrich, who then invited him to teach residents and see retina cases at UTMB. As Ruiz recalled, "After I had been there about three months, Dr. Gingrich said, 'Let's go have a cup of coffee.' While we were sitting in the cafeteria drinking coffee, he said, 'Dick, why don't you come down here full-time? Why don't you take over this department?'" By now Ruiz was deeply committed to staying in Houston and felt that he could not accept the offer of becoming a professor and chair of ophthalmology at UTMB. "He asked me to come down there full-time, and I have often wondered how different my life would have been if I would have done that. So anyway, things developed and I got very involved in the training program here at Hermann."[5]

Despite his grueling work schedule, Ruiz was deeply committed to the Hermann Hospital intern and resident training programs. "When I came back here, I immediately started getting involved in the training program which was, at that time, pretty meager," said Ruiz. "I found that I thoroughly enjoyed teaching, so I got more involved in it." Since the ophthalmology residency program was purely clinical, with no lecture series or didactics, Ruiz gradually introduced lectures and developed a more academic training program. His work there, along with his increasing renown as a retinal surgeon and general ophthalmologist, had a tremendous impact on the flow and number of patients, as well as the very nature of the ophthalmology training itself. Until 1961, eye surgery at Hermann Hospital was combined with the ear, nose, and throat (ENT) department. But around this time, the hospital's ophthalmology service began to schedule the use of an operating room independent of ENT. The number of patients scheduled for eye surgery increased to some twenty-five per week, and after Ruiz came to the hospital, it increased further. Lois Marie Dansdill Jr., a former ophthalmology nurse at Hermann, and Gayle Hodges, who also was on the nursing staff, recalled, "It wasn't until Dr. Ruiz came that we began to expand. They began to try to bring people in to help teach the residents. We went from being a small little eye hospital, or eye department, to a school."[6]

One of the residents at the time, Dr. Harry "Tom" Youens, who did both an internship and an ophthalmology residency at Hermann Hospital during the mid-1960s, remembered the impact that Dick Ruiz made on the teaching program. "He came on, I guess, about my last year at Hermann ... and Dick probably in one year taught as much to the residents as anybody else did in three years."[7]

Soon Ruiz also began working at M. D. Anderson Cancer Center. Dr. Thomas Royce, chief of ophthalmology at Hermann Hospital, ran the eye service for M. D. Anderson Cancer Center with the help of his private practice partner, Dr. Ralph Berkeley. But, as often happens in professional relationships, Royce and Berkeley separated sometime in late 1963 or early 1964. As Ruiz explained, "When they split up, Royce was the chief over at Anderson and the chief here [Hermann Hospital]. Anderson did not want to let Berkeley go, so they divided the service." This meant that for six months out of the year, Royce took care of the eye service at M. D. Anderson, and six months out of the year, Berkeley took care of it. Royce asked Ruiz to help him at Anderson and he began seeing patients in Royce's place, generally two half-day shifts per week,

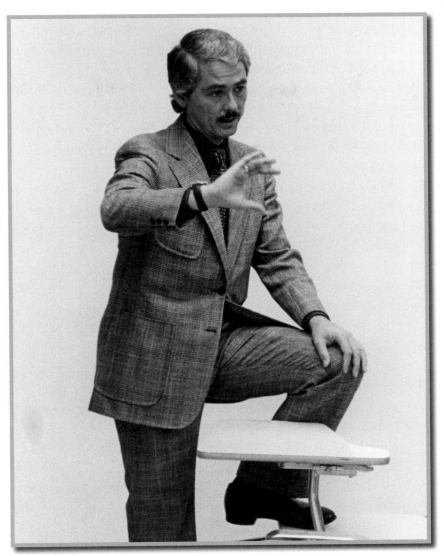

Dr. Ruiz teaching at UT Medical School, Houston.

on a voluntary basis. Berkeley's own ophthalmology practice was growing and, tiring of the demands imposed by the work at M. D. Anderson, he decided to step down. Dr. Royce then asked Ruiz to take over the responsibility of running the M. D. Anderson program. Ruiz accepted the challenging assignment and would fulfill this role for the next forty years. In November 1966, shortly after all of this transpired, the fifty-two-year-old Dr. Thomas Royce died unexpectedly from heart disease.[8]

Dr. Royce's sudden death shocked the medical community, and especially the doctors and staff in the eye service. Dr. Leigh Crozier, Hermann Hospital's executive director, now had the difficult task of recommending to the Hermann Hospital Estate board of trustees a replacement for Royce as chief of the service. Several doctors on staff had the seniority to take over as chief of the ophthalmology service. But Dr. Ruiz's dedication to teaching and his deep commitment to Hermann Hospital had not gone unnoticed by Dr. Crozier. Although Ruiz, at age thirty-five, was relatively young for the position and had been at Hermann for just four years, Crozier began seriously to consider naming him as the new chief of ophthalmology. Dr. Robert Stewart, a resident at the time, and who later joined Ruiz's group practice, recalled that "in fact, Dr. Crozier asked the residents who they wanted to be chief. There were some older guys that really wanted it, but they wanted it more for the prestige and were not ever that active in teaching. And Dick had already demonstrated a real desire to teach. So, we voted to have him become the chief."[9]

On January 16, 1967, the hospital formally announced Ruiz's appointment in a letter from Dr. A. Louis Dippel, Chief of Staff, and Dr. Leigh J. Crozier, Director, Hermann Hospital, to the medical staff of the ophthalmology section. In the letter, Dippel and Crozier asked the doctors to give Ruiz "their support and assistance" as he took on the new responsibilities. They also expressed their desire that the "service of Ophthalmology and the related educational program ... reach for many new goals right now and in the future."[10] Clearly, Hermann Hospital's administrators and its board of trustees had high expectations for the new chief of ophthalmology. They wanted someone who would devote the time and energy to the administrative functions required to run "a very active service," and who also would attract "top ranking residents" into the ophthalmology training program. Although

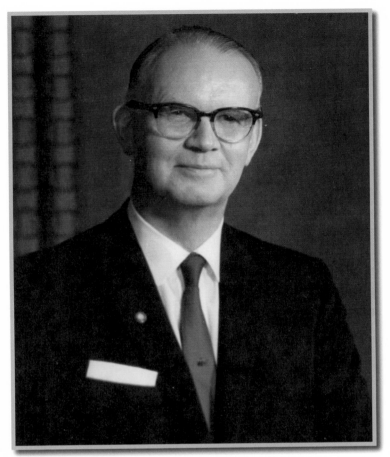

Leigh J. Crozier, MD, Director, Hermann Hospital, 1949-68.

the hospital offered no remuneration of any kind with the position—only the title "Chief of Service" and all the responsibility that came with it—Ruiz readily accepted the position. As a result of Ruiz's appointment, a few of the older doctors, having been passed over for the position, left Hermann to pursue their medical practices at other local hospitals.

"It was a very busy eye service," said Ruiz. "At that time, when Dr. Royce died in 1966, there were, as I recall, three residents—all good ones, too. So, with that as a basis, we built the program and it got better and better every year. And by the time the [University of Texas] medical school came here in 1970 . . . it was certainly one of the best training programs in the hospital." At the time, Hermann Hospital offered training programs in other areas including general surgery, urology, OB/GYN, and orthopedics, and had affiliation agreements with Baylor College of Medicine for internal medicine, ENT, and pediatrics.[11]

Dick Ruiz brought many changes to the hospital's ophthalmology training program. Several doctors who were residents during Ruiz's early years as chief of ophthalmology later shared their observations and recollections. Dr. George Gilbert Pyle Jr., had been an intern and resident, and for two years was on the medical staff at Hermann Hospital prior to Ruiz's arrival. He observed, "The Hermann program was fortunate that it had someone there [Ruiz] who was familiar with it and interested in taking over the training program. And it took off from there. It really took off." According to Pyle, the role of Dr. Leigh Crozier in fostering the development of the eye department at Hermann Hospital also should not be overlooked. "His interest in the department and the clinic was an important part in the development of the eye program. He saw to it that the finances were there to add the equipment, and to increase the amount of time devoted to ophthalmology, not only in surgery, but as far as nursing assistance and so forth."[12]

Robert Stewart remembered that the earlier training was very informal, but once Ruiz became chief, things began to change. He felt that the eye program was weak in pathology until Ruiz arranged a rotation at Baylor College of Medicine with Dr. Milton Boniuk (and later Dr. Ramon Font). Stewart acknowledged that at times, Ruiz was a demanding instructor. "The timing [for him] to become chief was good, the program has grown and has a good reputation," said Stewart. "Dr. Ruiz could be real hard to get along with some times, but he is a wonderful guy and his big attribute is that he's real fair. He never jacks anybody around. He's hardheaded and opinionated, but he's fair."[13]

Drs. Robert Lowe and Sue Ellen Young recalled a strong emphasis on improving the academics and the level of profession-alism in the training program. Lowe was both an intern and a resident in the Hermann Hospital program during 1968–72, and recalled that Ruiz "... did a good deal to bring in visiting profes-sors and have grand rounds with them. He pushed us . . . on the academics," said Lowe. "I think the Hermann program really had . . . a good mix of academics and hands-on experience." Dr. Sue Ellen Young graduated from UTMB in 1969 and did her residency around the same time as Lowe. She noted that Dr. Ruiz could be tough on the residents and put a lot of pressure on them to excel. "He made us very compulsive about details, and I think for that reason, I'm a good doctor now. I think we also kept up with the literature because he would ask us questions, and we were ter-ribly embarrassed if we didn't know the answer. It was loosely structured, and yet, there was a lot of pressure to be good." Young also observed that Ruiz worked hard, and gave of his own time to help the residents. "I think for a man like him ... in private prac-tice, he gave up a lot of his time. [He] wanted to make sure that we did a good job ... the main plus from that program is that he made us good doctors. And he was a good doctor and a good role model."[14]

Within a span of about five years, Dick Ruiz built up a medi-cal practice, took on the responsibility as chief of ophthalmology at Hermann, and in 1967, also began bringing partners into his private practice. His plan was to assemble an exceptional group of fellowship-trained subspecialists who would practice general ophthalmology and also bring special expertise to enhance the training program at Hermann Hospital. This was the prototype for the development of Houston Eye Associates and what later would become the Hermann Eye Center. The first to join was Dr. Charles Russo, who had trained in the Hermann Hospital pro-gram and had completed a retina fellowship under Dr. Ruiz. "He conceived the idea of building a [group of subspecialists] but, at the same time, practicing general ophthalmology so that you wouldn't be doing the same thing all the time," said Russo. "I liked the idea, and I liked working with him. He was an excellent teacher, excellent surgeon. So, we decided to stay on together."[15] In the meantime, Ruiz continued seeing patients in Galveston every Friday. Here, at UTMB, he first became acquainted with Dr. Malcolm Mazow, who taught at the medical school and who also was the ophthalmologist at the Public Health Service Hospital in Galveston. "I became good friends with Malcolm and he used to ask me to stop by the Public Health Service and consult with him on cases," said Ruiz. "He was a very academically oriented guy. He was the second person in the group. He loved to teach and he was a good teacher. He was a good part of this program for many, many years." Like Ruiz and Russo, Mazow graduated from UTMB. He joined them in July 1968. "We worked hard," Mazow remembered. "We would take call for every ophthalmologist in town who didn't want to work on weekends, and we worked six days a week." Mazow noted that as the group expanded, "there was no competition among the doctors. We all did general ophthalmology but we all had a special interest. And that was Dr. Ruiz's idea—to bring in people who were willing to do general ophthalmology, but who had a special interest or special training or both."[16]

The following year, Ruiz, Russo, and Mazow added two more ophthalmologists, Drs. Robert Wilkins and Robert Stewart, and changed the organization of their group practice from a partnership to a corporate structure (professional association) under the name, Houston Eye Associates. Each of the associates had taken specialized training after their residencies that brought expertise in a variety of important subspecialties to Houston Eye Associates. Stewart had trained in glaucoma; Wilkins, Dick Ruiz's cousin, in ophthalmic plastic surgery; Russo in retina; Mazow was a pediatric ophthalmologist; and of course, Dick Ruiz specialized in retina. "So now, there were five of us. Every one of these people had fellowship training. And I had guided all these folks to bring them back as a super-trained group for the Hermann Hospital training program, but also for a group that could offer real excellence in practice." Dr. Jeffrey Lanier joined the group next, in 1973, bringing his expertise in cornea and external disease. "So, we had a really good nucleus of well-trained people."[17]

During the key years of the middle 1960s to the early 1970s, other events took place both within and outside of Ruiz's ophthalmology practice that would have long-lasting consequences. On July 30, 1965, President Lyndon B. Johnson signed Medicare into law. Congress had been debating the idea of universal health care since the Truman administration, but the issue never garnered enough congressional support to pass as legislation. President Johnson brought an expansive social agenda when he took office following the assassination of President John F. Kennedy in November 1963. Presented as an amendment to Social Security, Medicare and its companion Medicaid represented the forefront

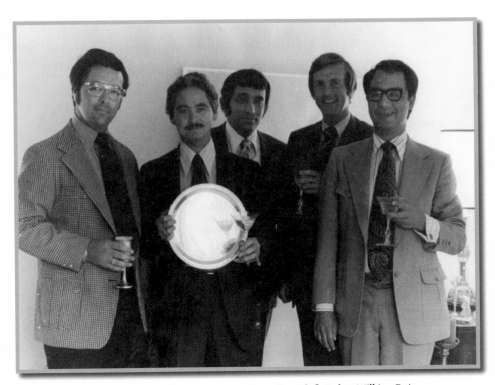

With Plate, *Richard Ruiz, founder, Houston Eye Associates. From left, Robert Wilkins, Ruiz, Malcolm Mazow, Robert Stewart, and Charles Russo.*

of Johnson's so-called Great Society and his War on Poverty. Simply put, Medicare offered two primary components: "Medicare Part A" provided a hospital insurance program for the elderly, and "Medicare Part B" created a voluntary supplementary medical insurance program. Medicaid, administered by the states, provided federal funds for medical care to the poor, primarily for low-income families with dependent children, the blind, and the disabled. Although many Americans feared the beginning of "socialized medicine," Johnson's overwhelming victory in the 1964 election brought many new liberals into the Congress who helped push the legislation. While both programs opened the door for better health care for the poor and the elderly, they also had an impact on the way doctors provided medical care and on the way teaching hospitals, including Hermann Hospital, functioned.

Prior to the passage of Medicare, medical interns and residents at Hermann Hospital had the benefit of treating and learning from a unique mix of patients, both charity "clinic" patients and private patients. Dr. Robert Lowe recalled how important the mix of indigent and paying patients was for the residents. "When I first started at Hermann, there was a very large clinic service," said Lowe. "I think that was kind of a unique thing. Most teaching hospitals are [either] all charity patients or all private patients. It wasn't a mix like we had. And this was made possible by the fact that Hermann was a privately endowed charity hospital. By the time I finished my residency, though, Medicare had gotten to a point where most patients [over age sixty-five] were private patients. And the system of having the charity hospital had changed a great deal just by the impact of Medicare in those four to five years." Medical education felt the impact of these changing patient demographics across the country, as did the private practice of medicine. The result was a change in the sense of both funded and unfunded patients being treated at both tax-supported and private teaching hospitals where medical residents could gain hands-on experience under the supervision of experienced practitioners.[18]

Dr. Malcolm Mazow also observed, "Prior to Medicare, there was a lot of really good care being done in [charity] hospitals. Medicare came in and changed a lot of that—not all good, but not all bad." What is clear is that Medicare wrought extensive changes in the lives of Americans, especially physicians, patients, and those engaged in all aspects of health care.[19]

Medicare notwithstanding, Dick Ruiz realized a continuing need for supplementary funding to enhance the Hermann Hospital eye service and to provide additional funds for treating indigent patients who were not eligible for Medicare. During the spring of 1968, he created the Houston Eye Fund (its name was changed to Hermann Eye Fund in October 1980) with three primary goals in mind: to provide funds for research related to the eye; to provide care for indigent patients with serious eye problems; and to provide teaching in the field of ophthalmology. Ruiz's previous desire to practice general ophthalmology provided opportunities for him to treat a wide range of patients, and this large pool of personal contacts later enhanced his ability to conduct fundraising. During the next forty years, the Eye Fund grew to where it provided nearly $1 million annually in funding for hospital services (professional eye services were always donated) to indigent and semi-indigent patients, becoming part of an outreach program that included the San José Clinic, Commission for the Blind, University of Houston School of Optometry, Lighthouse for the Blind, county health clinics, and community health agencies in Baytown, Acres Home, Settegast, and the Harris County Hospital District's Lyndon B. Johnson General Hospital. The Fund helps patients who are uninsured and who may "fall between the cracks" of Medicare and Medicaid coverage.

Other developments during this time would also have an impact on Ruiz's private practice and his work at Hermann. Rumors circulated for several years across Texas about the creation of one or more new medical schools to help meet the state's increasing demand for more physicians. Finally, in May 1969, the Texas legislature passed a bill authorizing the creation of a new medical school in Houston. Two weeks later, on June 13, 1969, in the auditorium of the Jesse H. Jones Library Building in the Texas Medical Center, Gov. Preston Smith signed the bill creating The University of Texas Medical School at Houston. This move caused some controversy, since a medical school—Baylor College of Medicine—already existed in Houston's Texas Medical Center. But statewide, Texas needed more medical doctors, and Houston was only one of the cities that would be home to new medical schools during the next decade. Additionally, the legislature voted to provide a medical school at Texas Tech University in Lubbock (coincidentally, Governor Smith's hometown) and tax-supported funding for Baylor College of Medicine, ensuring that the school's enrollment would not be adversely affected due to its difference in tuition with the state school. Dr. Charles LeMaistre, who held numerous positions—from professor to chancellor—in The University of Texas System during his long career, recalled years later, "There was much concern as to whether this would hurt Baylor very badly." Officials from The University of Texas system pledged not to recruit full-time faculty from Baylor Medical School, and that they would not contravene any of Baylor's teaching contracts with other hospitals. "Additionally, we worked closely with the Hermann Estate, Hermann Hospital, and the Texas Medical Center," said LeMaistre. "Finding the best way to do it resulted in a lot of compromises, but the compromises turned out to be very worthwhile." One of the keys to locating a new medical school in Houston stemmed from the willingness of the Hermann Hospital Estate board of trustees, some of whom (notably Walter Sterling and Jack Josey) served on the Board of Regents of The University of Texas, to have the hospital serve as the primary teaching hospital for the new medical school. LeMaistre stated that "Hermann Hospital stepping forward and offering to be the primary teaching hospital was the key."[20]

Indeed, the late 1960s became a critical time for Hermann Hospital. It had been twenty years since the opening of the "new" building (later known as the Corbin J. and Wilhelmina C. Robertson Pavilion), and some of the facilities were showing signs of wear. During this time, Methodist Hospital flourished in its role as the primary hospital for the Baylor faculty's private patients, but provided no indigent care, while Hermann Hospital began to languish. The city-county hospitals, Jefferson Davis Hospital and the recently opened (1963) Ben Taub Hospital, were used as the primary teaching hospitals for Baylor medical students, interns, and residents. When officials first announced that Hermann would be the primary teaching hospital for the new University of Texas Medical School, the medical staff anticipated that the new arrangement might help rejuvenate the hospital. But Dick Ruiz recalled that once the new relationship had been confirmed and plans were being laid for the new medical school, Hermann's medical staff began to have second thoughts. "Now, we had an opportunity to get 'our' medical school and everybody was very excited about it. But then when it came right down to the medical school coming and Hermann Hospital was to be the main teaching hospital, the medical staff started getting concerned about the medical school's full-time faculty taking over the hospital—and [worrying that] the guys who had been working here for years would be left in the cold."[21]

Although accounts differ, evidence suggests that a change in the original affiliation agreement between the Hermann Hospital Estate and The University of Texas Board of Regents was the catalyst for what happened next. On November 15, 1967, The University of Texas Regents, the Hermann Hospital Trustees, and medical staff leaders from the hospital met to examine a proposed affiliation agreement. Prior to this, Hermann Hospital had two main committees: the education committee, comprised of the chiefs of services that had training programs; and the executive committee, including the hospital director, chief of staff, secretary, and three appointees from the medical staff. All committees reported to the executive committee. A primary concern for the medical staff was that the proposed affiliation agreement would replace the hospital's executive committee with a medical board that would control the quality of patient care. The new education committee was to be comprised of the chairs of all the clinical departments in the medical school. All of the hospital's committees would report to the medical board, which included the "Hermann Hospital director, the chief-of-staff, staff secretary, and five members elected by the medical staff." The hospital's medical staff would be in the majority on this new board. With this system in place, in which the medical staff held sway on the medical board and the medical school's department chairs controlled the education committee, the medical staff was comfortable enough with the new division of authority to agree to the affiliation agreement. The final agreement, dated January 1, 1968, included "two common objectives agreed upon between the UT Board of Regents and Hermann Hospital Estate: teaching and research sought primarily by the university, and care of patients and community services sought primarily by the hospital."[22]

Historian Bryant Boutwell wrote in his book, *Conversation with a Medical School*, that "There are many variations to the story regarding the unhappiness generated among a number of the Hermann Hospital private-practice physicians, but all revolve around the central theme of Medical School clinical department heads creating a potential layer of control over private physicians that would not be tolerated." In June 1970, an ad hoc Committee chaired by Dr. L. Rodney Rodgers discovered that "our concept of the Executive Board and the Medical Education Board [were] so different from the version that we had studied in November 1967." The committee was "dumbfounded by the changes made to the Medical Board composition. It now combined both the Executive and Education Committees into one dictatorial committee." This meant that the executive committee of the medical staff would no longer have a Hermann Hospital majority. "We were concerned that this second layer of authority over the private physicians would deter our traditional access to our governing Board of Trustees," said Rodgers. The doctors believed that this arrangement would do away with their control over patient care.

In addition, of approximately 860 physicians on staff at the time (one-third of whom were regular staff; two-thirds courtesy staff), hospital director Dan G. Kadrovach believed that only about 125 of the doctors had both the enthusiasm for teaching and the willingness to sacrifice the time away from their medical practices to devote to students. Thus, the changing authority system was even more onerous to the doctors who had no desire to become involved in teaching at the new medical school. Ultimately, the issues surrounding the affiliation agreement would not be resolved until 1987, when Edward Randall III became chair of the board of the Hermann Hospital Estate and insisted on a new affiliation agreement with The University of Texas.[23]

While this controversy continued to fester, the Hermann Hospital Estate's board of trustees approved construction of a new building, to be known as the Jesse H. Jones Pavilion, to accommodate the needs of the new medical school. Newly appointed hospital director Kadrovach found himself in the center of an embroiling situation which would prove pivotal to the future of Hermann Hospital. On the one hand, it was a moment of great opportunity to restore some of the luster to the hospital in its new role as the teaching hospital for The University of Texas Medical School. On the other hand, it was a moment of economic peril as well, since the financial obligations for the new building were significant. Due to this tight financial situation and as a means of cutting construction costs, hospital officials decided that there was no immediate need for additional bed space. Therefore, they would build out only six of the planned eight floors in the new building. Floors seven and eight would remain "shells" until some future time when the need for space justified the expense of finishing out the remaining areas. Ultimately the Jones Pavilion would be a ten-story structure, including a designated ground level and the 1978 addition of a ninth floor with clay tile parapet roof structures.[24]

As all of this transpired, The University of Texas took a major step in January 1970, when the Board of Regents announced the appointment of Dr. Cheves M. Smythe as dean of the new Houston medical school. The Harvard-trained Smythe had an impressive résumé, and at the time of his appointment he was associate director of the Association of American Medical Colleges with a faculty appointment at Northwestern School of Medicine. The new dean faced an enormous task: to build a medical school from scratch and at the same time to bring together the operations of Hermann Hospital and the school. Smythe recalled the sense of urgency during the early days of the UT medical school: "When one has students staring down his throat, no faculty, no facilities—you've got to get things done." Smythe had concerns of his own about the hospital. "In the late 1960s, Hermann Hospital, which had had a proud record ... had fallen on hard times. The notion was that the medical school would do something about

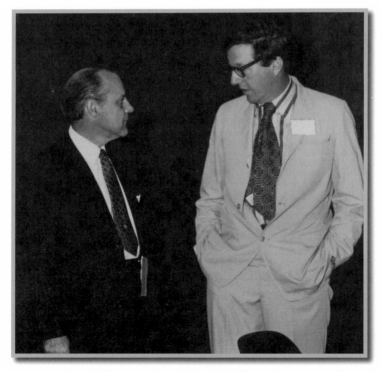

Dan G. Kadrovach, director, Hermann Hospital, 1968-75; Cheves M. Smythe, MD, founding dean, The University of Texas Medical School, Houston, 1970-75.

that." Hermann Hospital's Dan Kadrovach and Dean Cheves Smythe began to work out the details of the new relationship. As Ruiz observed, "You can imagine the immensity of trying to bring a medical school into being and to marry it to a hospital that really never had been an academic institution, even though we had some residency training programs. I don't know many people that could have done that except Cheves Smythe. It took that kind of fortitude and intelligence and understanding of not only the academics and the medical school but the interface with the hospital and the clinical side of it."[25]

Ruiz knew that the coming of the medical school meant that the university's department chairs would replace the chiefs of the services in the hospital. The university system required that the professors work on a full-time basis and under the practice guidelines established by the university. This meant that Ruiz might have to give up his private practice if he wished to have an academic appointment and continue as chief of the eye service in the hospital—something he was unwilling to do. Consequently, he submitted his resignation as chief of ophthalmology to Dan Kadrovach. As much as he wanted a faculty appointment, Ruiz had no interest in being in a full-time system with the attendant tethers and bureaucracy. Both Kadrovach and Smythe were stunned by his resignation. He had been with Hermann for some ten years and been chief of ophthalmology for about four years. During his tenure, the intern and resident training programs improved significantly. Ruiz was the obvious and natural first choice to head the ophthalmology program in the new medical school.

Smythe and Kadrovach requested a meeting, as Ruiz recalled years later. He told them that he knew that The University of Texas had a full-time system, and that he did not want to serve in that capacity. His desire was to continue his private practice, work out of Hermann Hospital, and to step aside so they could appoint a full-time chairman for the position. But Kadrovach and Smythe did not want Ruiz to quit, not only because they felt he could do the job but also because he was already on-site and would cost both institutions almost nothing. They asked what it would take for him to stay as chief of ophthalmology. Ruiz stated that he did not want a salary or tenure. What he wanted was a measure of autonomy and independence that was essentially unheard of in academe. He told them, "I want you to make it [ophthalmology] a department. I won't do it as a division (subset) of surgery. Then, I want you to let me run it and, of course, you have every right to replace me if you are not satisfied with what I am doing, and that is fine. I don't want any contract. If you are not happy with me, you should ask me to leave and I will." Kadrovach and Smythe agreed to accept Ruiz's offer and to take it to their respective boards for final approval.[26]

In March 1971, Richard Ruiz became among the first to receive academic appointments at the new medical school. Evidence suggests that Dr. William Fields, a neurologist, likely received the first clinical faculty appointment. Dr. Fields was the only neurologist in the southwest when he came to Houston in 1949. He established the neurology services at both the Veteran's Hospital and at Hermann Hospital, and became chair of the neurology department at Baylor College of Medicine. He moved to the Southwestern Medical School in Dallas in 1967, but returned to Houston in 1969 after being appointed to the faculty of the new University of Texas Medical School. He recalled that Dr. Ruiz's part-time appointment caused a stir among some at the medical school.

> He was already on the scene when the medical school came.
> He was quite logically the best candidate to head a department
> of ophthalmology. Sure, there were some objections, but
> these objections came largely from some of the newcomers
> to the scene who felt that academia needed to be "pure" and
> that to have somebody who was an entrepreneur—and I
> think that we all know that Dr. Ruiz is an entrepreneur, and
> a good one—they kind of frowned on that. But I think they
> were clearly persuaded by some of us who saw that there

was virtue in doing it the other way. But the Department of
Ophthalmology still is unique in this regard. All the other
units of the medical school are headed by full-time persons. I
have nothing but admiration for Dr. Ruiz. He pulled it off![27]

While Dick Ruiz was enthusiastic about the impending opening
of the new medical school and his appointment as a department
chairman, many of his colleagues at Hermann Hospital continued to have reservations about the affiliation agreement. It is not
clear who first proposed the idea, but in 1972, six of the doctors
who were on the medical staff of Hermann Hospital and who
were frustrated by the changing administrative structure vis-à-vis
the medical school decided that they would build their own hospital. Their decision likely was influenced by the fact that during
this time, doctor-owned hospitals were proving to be very lucrative. The original group quickly expanded to include twenty-two
general partners and some 125 limited partners in the venture.
The new 356-bed, doctor-owned Park Plaza Hospital opened
three years later on April 13, 1975. "About the time that the medical school came, there was sort of a mass exodus of those old-
time medical staff members who had supported this hospital for
a long time with big practices and paying patients," said Dick
Ruiz. Losing many of the longtime medical staff meant the loss
of those doctors' patients, a large portion of Hermann Hospital's
"client base." The timing for such a venture, however, was good
from the doctors' perspective, since Medicare developed into a
major source of funds for doctors and hospitals who now treated patients that were previously charity cases or had no access
to health care at all. Now, the Park Plaza doctors could maintain
their autonomy without worrying about the medical school faculty imposing standards and taking over their hospital. They had a
high chance for financial success because they already maintained
large medical practices, and Medicare/Medicaid helped pay for
many of their patients' professional and hospital services.[28]

Despite the continuing controversy with Hermann Hospital,

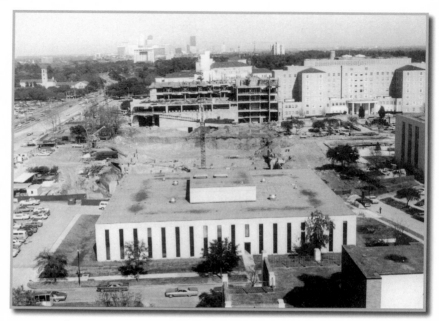

Foreground, UT Medical School's John Freeman Building; Center, construction crane for UT Medical School main building; Background, unfinished Jones Pavilion.

Dean Smythe continued his efforts to build a faculty and develop plans for the new medical school. Smythe labored over stacks of forms and secured a federal grant to help fund building construction. The first nineteen students, who enrolled in 1970, initially attended classes in San Antonio, Dallas, and Galveston before settling in at various locations in the Texas Medical Center. In June 1971, the medical school welcomed the first thirty-two students who would complete all of their studies in Houston. Two months later, construction began on the school's first structure, the two-story, 55,000-square-foot John H. Freeman Building. Once the Freeman Building opened in August 1972, The University of Texas Medical School at Houston had a physical "home" in the Texas Medical Center. With a faculty in place and construction on the large (851,818 square feet) Medical School Building and the Jones Pavilion of Hermann Hospital underway, the new medical school was a reality.[29]

Dick Ruiz looked back on that time and recalled, "Cheves just kind of let me run with it. I didn't do anything different. We already had a training program and I had five associates. And we all had busy practices. Every one of the associates had an extra year of training in a subspecialty so we were a very well-trained group—perfect for an academic clinical program. And so, things rolled along there for three or four years." Sometime during 1973 or early 1974, as construction on the Jones Pavilion was underway, Ruiz began to think seriously about a concept that he had been developing for some time. The seventh floor of the new Jones Pavilion at Hermann Hospital, left unfinished, was still uncommitted. To Ruiz, this presented a unique opportunity. His idea was to create a world-class eye center built upon an enhanced version of the clinical practice he founded and its relationship to the teaching program in Hermann Hospital. The model included the department of ophthalmology in The University of Texas Medical School, and melded it with the intern and resident training programs at the hospital and with the highly trained doctors in his clinical practice at Houston Eye Associates. "It was only after Dr. Ruiz's position as a chairman on a part-time basis had become solidified that he was then able to proceed with getting the Eye Center put together," said Dr. William Fields. "And it was certainly a year or a year and a half after that before the Eye Center was more than just something in his mind's eye."[30]

Although Ruiz did not specifically create his model for the Hermann Eye Center based upon any other eye centers in the country, his years in residency at Wayne State University under Dr. A. D. Ruedemann and his fellowship with Dr. Charles Schepens at Harvard did have a profound influence on how he decided to organize it. He admired both men's independent spirit and particularly Schepens' organizational skills and entrepreneurial bent. "Schepens had a sort of free enterprise, wheeler-dealer approach," Ruiz recalled. "He avoided the bureaucracy of an institution—the bureaucratic processes of it—which could be very hampering. I observed that and it stuck in my mind ... I learned a lot, watching him." Ruiz formulated a clear idea of how he wanted to set up the Eye Center in terms of its organization, its relationship with the hospital and the medical school, and even its physical design. "I'd been in private practice long enough to know how I wanted this thing to operate from a flow standpoint. I wanted it to operate like a private practice, not like some clinic or some private institution. I ... wanted to apply what I'd learned in [my] years of private practice to the design of the place. The indigent patient care concept—how to handle that—was strictly mine." Dick Ruiz also knew that the key to success was fulfilling the needs and responsibilities for both Hermann Hospital and UT–Houston, and both institutions needed easy and unencumbered exits if they were not satisfied.[31]

Ruiz developed his plan to the last detail, including how to fund the indigent care program, which he proposed to take over from the hospital in exchange for space in the new building, and the mechanics of how the eye center would interact with the hospital. He knew that the seventh floor of the new Jones Pavilion was empty and not scheduled to be built out. Late in 1973, he engaged the services of the Rice University Department of Architecture's Rice Health Facilities Studio Team to create a plan that included his innovative ideas for an ophthalmology treatment and teaching center. After an extensive series of meetings, surveys, and planning sessions, in the spring of 1974, the Health Facilities Studio Team presented Ruiz with a seventy-nine page, comprehensive plan, *Ophthalmology Center*.[32] The booklet, complete with floor plans, drawings, photographs, and flowcharts, provided a resource that Ruiz could use in his campaign to gain approval from the hospital trustees and the medical school administration. "And so, that is when I went to the Hermann Hospital Estate board of trustees. This was probably around 1973 or 1974," he recalled, "and asked them if I could build an eye center up here on the seventh floor if I could raise the money to build out the floor." Ruiz's proposal was highly unusual since it included a for-profit private practice as one of the components in a mainly non-profit world. But he was convinced that this idea would be of benefit to the hospital, the medical school, the patients, and to the staff. Here was a unique opportunity to take three separate entities with an established relationship and create a showcase program that would benefit all by pulling them closer together through this proposed Hermann Eye Center.[33]

The hospital's trustees were intrigued with the idea and, after some serious salesmanship by Dick Ruiz, indicated their tentative support for his proposal and authorized him to raise up to $1 million to provide initial funds for the project. After all, he would provide eye care for the indigent patients of the hospital in return for use of the empty space on the seventh floor of the new building, and he would pay all the expenses for the build-out and furnishings. But before he began raising the money to pay for the new facilities, Ruiz wanted to be certain that the medical school was fully on board with his plan. "That is when I went to Cheves Smythe and told him, 'I've got the trustees of the Hermann Hospital Estate to agree to let me build an eye center on the seventh floor of the Jones Pavilion if I can raise the money to do it, and I want the blessing of The University of Texas so that this can be the service arm, the clinical arm, for the department of ophthalmology. And I don't want to do it unless I have that blessing.'" As Smythe recalled years later, "Here one had an energetic guy, a native Houstonian, a graduate of the Galveston medical school [UTMB], trained at the Hermann Hospital, very loyal to it, wanting to develop ophthalmology..." Smythe seemed agreeable to the notion and, with his hands full with other issues related to the medical school, felt that it was a strong plan that immediately benefited and enhanced the department of ophthalmology without costing any money.

But the approval for the eye center was not yet formalized. Ruiz needed to overcome opposition from several of the medical school's department chairs and faculty in order to implement his plan. With the initial approval of the hospital's board of trustees and the support of the dean, the chances for Ruiz getting formal approval from the medical school for his concept looked promising. He was counting on Dean Cheves Smythe's endorsement to help convince those on the full-time faculty who had doubts or who opposed his plan.[34]

However, an unanticipated turn of events proved that gaining this approval would not be easy. In March 1975, Dr. Charles Berry, president of the recently constituted University of Texas Health Science Center at Houston, unexpectedly fired Dean Smythe. The Health Science Center had been created in 1972, under acting president Dr. John Victor Olsen, as an organizational umbrella that included all of the university's Houston medical branches except the M. D. Anderson Cancer Center. Smythe later recalled that, having the choice of resigning or being fired, he told Berry to fire him. "That way, Dr. Berry would have to do the explaining, not me," said Smythe. Loquacious by nature, Smythe also had great insight into bureaucracies and institutions, and he knew the value of silence; he would let the record speak for itself. But his dismissal as dean suddenly placed Ruiz's plan for a comprehensive, world-class eye center in jeopardy of being seriously delayed, if not cancelled altogether. Although he was no longer dean of the medical school, Smythe remained a highly productive member of the faculty, practicing medicine and teaching. Years later, Ruiz recalled, "Cheves continued full-time as professor of medicine and subsequently won several Best Teacher awards. He played a key teaching role at Lyndon Baines Johnson Hospital over the years and continued to provide exceptional medical consultative services for my private patients. And twenty years later, in 1995, The University of Texas Health Science Center once again turned to Cheves and asked him to serve as dean pro tem following Dr. John Ribble's decision to step down."

Along with the loss of a key ally in Dean Smythe, other challenges simmering in the background began to come to a boil, and Ruiz faced what appeared to be insurmountable problems in bringing his idea for an eye center to fruition. The main challenge was to convince the new administration—from President Berry to the new dean, Robert Tuttle—and subsequently the medical school faculty, to approve his plan for the Eye Center. He also had to keep the board of trustees of the Hermann Hospital Estate from wavering as well. The months ahead would be a major test of Dick Ruiz's persuasive powers and his patience, with no guarantee of success.

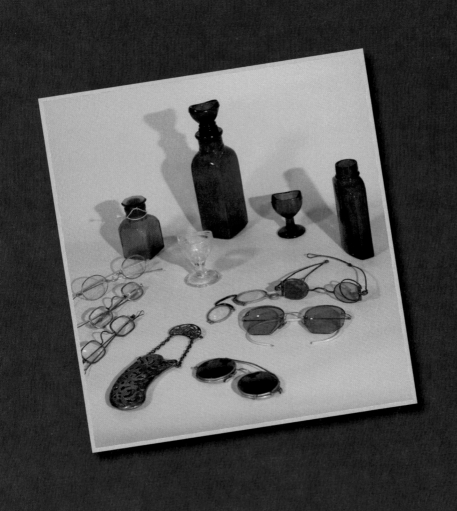

CHAPTER FOUR

Challenges & Diverging Paths

T HE FIRING OF the medical school's founding dean, Cheves M. Smythe, in March 1975, left Dick Ruiz without an important ally and the proposed eye center in very precarious circumstances. The idea of building a world-class eye center and bringing together the best elements of a teaching hospital, medical school, and the private practice of ophthalmology was both innovative and bold. But it also was an idea that was complex and controversial. In order to gain final approval from all of the institutions and departments involved with the proposed eye center, Dick Ruiz had to wage a multi-faceted campaign with the medical school, its new Health Science Center umbrella administration, the Hermann Hospital Estate board of trustees, and the hospital's CEO. The chain of events that finally led to the establishment of the Hermann Eye Center and its subsequent history over the next fifteen years provides a clear illustration of the challenges involved with bringing a medical school, a teaching hospital, and private practice physicians together in one overarching endeavor.

Shortly after Smythe's dismissal as dean, the hospital's board of trustees asked Ruiz, by "special invitation," to present his full proposal during their meeting on April 1, 1975. Ruiz talked in detail about his idea, and by this time he also had the initial plans from the Rice Department of Architecture's Health Facilities Stu-

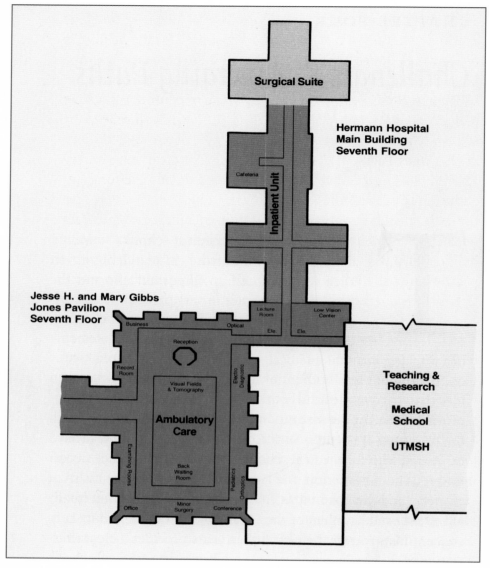

Hermann Eye Center's original design included the seventh floors of the interconnected Main Building (Robertson Pavilion), Jones Pavilion, and the UT Medical School.

dio Team (also referred to as the Rice Design Alliance), to use as a vivid illustration of his proposal. Plans called for the hospital's new Jesse H. Jones Pavilion to be physically connected with the medical school's main building, which was to be constructed in such a manner that the two buildings would be contiguous. Ruiz's plan proposed to take advantage of this construction scheme by locating the ophthalmology outpatient clinic on the seventh floor of the Jones Pavilion, the ophthalmology surgical suite on the seventh floor of the hospital's interconnected main building (renamed the Corbin J. and Wilhelmina C. Robertson Pavilion), and the department of ophthalmology offices and basic research labs on the interconnected seventh floor of the new medical school building. This validated the use of the term "center," denoting a place where patients, faculty, staff, and students could move easily from one component of the Eye Center to another.

During this meeting with the trustees, Ruiz indicated that he already had raised some $200,000 and affirmed that he would build out the outpatient part of the eye service. Originally, he planned to dedicate about half of the space to inpatient beds and reserve half for outpatient services. But by the mid-1970s, eye doctors were performing more and more surgical procedures on an outpatient basis. In addition, with the opening of Park Plaza hospital, a number of doctors had left Hermann, which made more beds available. Thus, Ruiz felt that Hermann Hospital already had sufficient bed space for inpatient procedures and modified his plans to reflect the emphasis on developing an outpatient center. Ruiz stated that he would use Hermann Hospital for all inpatient procedures and that he wanted "complete operational control" of the eye center, including billing and collecting. He reiterated that he did not plan to join The University of Texas Medical School as a full-time faculty member, but would prefer to serve as part-time faculty. He also offered to help in the search should the university require a full-time chairman for the ophthalmology department. After a lengthy discussion following Ruiz's presentation, the board instructed the hospital's director, Dan Kadrovach, and the executive director of the Hermann Hospital Estate, Neill Amsler, to set up a meeting with Dr. Charles Berry, president of The University of Texas Health Science Center at Houston (UTHSC–H), to discuss Ruiz's proposal and then report back to the board. Dr. Charles "Chuck" Berry, the former medical director at the Johnson Space Center, had been appointed president of the newly created UTHSC–H in 1974.[1]

During this time, as the medical school was becoming established in the Texas Medical Center, the dean had begun holding regular monthly meetings with the department chairmen. In one of these meetings an ad hoc committee of medical school department chairpersons was formed to review Ruiz's proposed eye center and make a recommendation to the group. The committee was created at Ruiz's request by Dr. Robert Tuttle, who succeeded Cheves Smythe as dean of the Medical School. Also appointed to the committee was Dan Kadrovach, CEO of Hermann Hospital. This committee was put together to discuss and establish the interrelationship of the Hermann Eye Center to Hermann Hospital and The University of Texas Medical School. Dr. William S. Fields, chair of the department of neurology, headed the committee and recalled that they debated "long and hard" over the main issue, which was that Dr. Ruiz would not be a full-time faculty member and that he would be department chairperson (called program director at that time) in the medical school and also continue to work in private practice, outside of the university's "practice plan."[2]

During the weeks and months that the ad hoc committee conducted its deliberations, Ruiz made two appearances before the medical school's faculty senate to discuss his proposal and answer questions. As the process dragged on, an additional complication developed when Dan Kadrovach resigned as Hermann Hospital's director on August 1, 1975, apparently after a disagreement with the board of trustees over funding allocations to meet the needs of the new hospital-medical school affiliation.[3]

In September, the department heads met again and Fields reported on the ad hoc committee's findings. As Dick Ruiz recalled,

Dr. Rod Howell, chair of Pediatrics, moved that the group endorse the planned eye center. "I don't remember who seconded it but they unanimously endorsed the concept of letting me develop an eye center," Ruiz said. "And the thing that really sold the full-time academics was when I said 'I don't want tenure and I don't want any money.' So, once I said I didn't want any tenure, there was a collective sigh of relief." Fields noted that Ruiz could have created an eye center that had nothing to do with the medical school or he could have abandoned the idea of having the eye center in the hospital and developed a clinic in the medical school. "So the two things really had to mesh," said Fields. "It was a very skillful job that Dr. Ruiz did in convincing both sides that this was to everybody's advantage."[4]

But despite this vote of confidence, Ruiz still did not have a definitive answer regarding his proposal. He wrote to the board of trustees of the Hermann Hospital Estate on October 3, 1975, and politely but firmly presented an ultimatum. "I will stand on my past record as a steadfast and loyal supporter and more recently as a defender of Hermann Hospital," Ruiz began. He reviewed that many months before he had presented his proposal to develop a comprehensive ophthalmology program. He stated that on September 17, the administrative council of the medical school, which included all of the program chairs, "unanimously endorsed the proposal," but since receiving this endorsement, he had "heard nothing from the Hermann Board and nothing from the Medical School" regarding the Eye Center. It seemed that perhaps, because of the administrative turnover, no one was willing or able to take action regarding the ophthalmology program. He reiterated that he had done everything possible to help the hospital and felt that he had exhausted every avenue. "Gentlemen, I have done everything in my power and, in fact, have exceeded the limits of good judgment in my efforts to exert a positive influence on Hermann's plight. I personally cannot tolerate the lack of direction or positive thinking as concerns the Ophthalmology Program. If by November 1, 1975, I do not have a full endorsement of the Board to proceed with negotiations both with the hospital and The University of Texas Medical School at Houston to pursue the objective previously outlined to you, I will have to assume you are not interested."[5]

Ruiz's ultimatum seems finally to have overcome the inertia on the part of the Hermann Hospital Estate board of trustees. At their next meeting on October 21, 1975, the Hermann Hospital Estate executive director, Neill Amsler, reviewed for the trustees the history of Ruiz's proposal. The trustees asked Amsler and Dr. Charles Berry for an update on the "current status" of this proposition. Berry stated that Ruiz "conferred twice with the Medical Staff Faculty Senate, following which the Senate voted to recommend approval of his proposal, although there were some reservations." They then instructed Dan Kadrovach's newly appointed successor, William Smith, to schedule "an early meeting with Dr. Ruiz," and also suggested that Dr. Berry do the same, "in order to finalize arrangements for implementation of Dr. Ruiz' proposal." Berry assured the board that "a meeting will be held involving himself and Messrs. Amsler, Smith, Doctors Tuttle and Ruiz, in this regard in the near future."[6]

Tuttle informed Ruiz of this last hurdle and arranged the meeting. As Ruiz remembered, "We were sitting around a little conference table ... Robert Tuttle, Ed McLaughlin, and one other person I do not remember." Tuttle introduced Ruiz, who recalled that "I told Dr. Berry that I wanted to make a world-class eye center, teach medical students and residents, and take good care of patients and help the hospital—I talked about thirty minutes. Dr. Berry did not interrupt me much at all; he just listened. When I got through, he looked over at Bob Tuttle, and said, 'Bob, it sounds like a great idea. Why don't you help him?'" With Berry's support in hand, the hospital's trustees could now give their unanimous support to Ruiz's proposed Eye Center. Finally, on December 2, 1975, the Hermann Hospital Estate Board of Trustees gave the go-ahead for which Ruiz had worked so long and hard. The minutes of that meeting reported, "Mr. Smith reviewed with the

Trustees the recent discussion held with Dr. Ruiz and requested that the Board endorse a proposal set forth by Dr. Ruiz to convert Hospital space on the Seventh Floor." In addition, the hospital's trustees unanimously agreed to help Ruiz with raising funds and contacting philanthropic foundations on his behalf.[7]

Most likely, the administrative turmoil at both the medical school and the hospital caused the trustees to take extra time considering the ramifications of approving the Center. As Ruiz recalled later, "I told the hospital, 'Look, if you let me build an eye center up there, I will take your indigent clinic off your hands and run it for you. You won't have to pay for anything. You won't have to hire anybody. I'll run it, I'll manage it, and we will do the indigent service which you are obligated to deliver.'" Ruiz asked to have the seventh floor of the Jones Pavilion on a rent-free basis, a trade-off for managing the hospital's eye clinic, providing services for the indigent patients, and raising the money to build out the floor. He pledged to use Hermann Hospital exclusively for surgery, for any patients who needed to be hospitalized, and for laboratory studies. This guaranteed eye patients and cash flow for the hospital. "In other words," said Ruiz, "we [would] support the hospital 100 percent. And so, they all agreed with that and that is the way it has been for all these years."[8]

Ruiz, with endorsements from the Hermann Hospital Estate Board of Trustees and the president of The University of Texas Health Science Center at Houston, continued his fundraising campaign with a new sense of urgency. Since opening his ophthalmology practice in Houston, Ruiz had treated or become acquainted with a number of prominent Houstonians, including George R. Brown, Corbin Robertson, and John H. Freeman, people to whom he now turned for financial support for the Eye Center. Knowing that he needed to explore all avenues, he also appealed to the Houston Endowment, the Cullen Foundation, the Brown Foundation, and the M. D. Anderson Foundation. As he remembered later, "Every one of them supported the fundraising effort." These four major foundations together contributed some $1 million to help launch the Hermann Eye Center. Over the years, these and other foundations, philanthropists, and individual donors have continued to generously support the Hermann Eye Center. Many people observed that Dick Ruiz possessed a unique ability to raise funds, but he also had a worthy cause—improved teaching, research, and patient care in ophthalmology—that people wanted to support.[9]

Early in 1977, as the build-out construction moved forward on the seventh floor of the Jones Pavilion, Dr. Berry resigned as president of The University of Texas Health Science Center. The University of Texas regents then turned to a legendary figure, Dr. Truman G. Blocker, to serve on an interim basis until they could conduct a search and appoint a permanent president. Blocker, an imposing figure at about six feet, four inches in height and weighing some 250 pounds, was highly regarded as a plastic surgeon, professor, chief of plastic surgery, and former president of UTMB, and was outspoken in his loyalty to The University of Texas. Ruiz was enthusiastic about the appointment and had great respect for Blocker. "He had become world famous because of the Texas City disaster," said Ruiz. On April 16, 1947, a ship containing over 2,300 tons of ammonium nitrate exploded while docked at Texas City, a seaport community between Houston and Galveston. The ensuing explosions resulted in approximately 581 killed, and over five thousand injured, making this possibly the worst industrial accident in American history. Blocker treated many who were badly burned in the explosions, becoming world-renowned as a burn expert in the process.[10]

Since the Hermann Eye Center had not yet opened, it was important for Ruiz to convince Blocker to support the project. During a committee meeting that Blocker attended, he told Ruiz in his usual, straightforward manner for all to hear, "I hear you are building an eye center over there, Ruiz. I want to see it." Following the meeting, Ruiz took Blocker on a tour and provided a detailed description of how the facility would function. The build-out was still underway, with drywall being installed and lots of dust and debris lying about, but it was possible to imagine how the center would look once the construction was finished. After Ruiz showed Blocker through the space, the two men paused at the window where the Jones Pavilion connected to the new medical school building. Ruiz wanted to be certain that Blocker understood his agreement with the hospital and the medical school. As he recalled later, "I thought, 'There is never going to be a better time to tell him.' I said, 'Dr. Blocker, you do realize that this is going to be run as a separate corporation?' He looked down at me and did not say a word for about thirty seconds. I thought, 'What is going to happen here?' And then he said, 'That is all right. We need a lot more of this.' That was all he said." In addition to granting his approval for the Eye Center, Blocker threw his personal endorsement behind Ruiz's fund raising efforts. "I was still trying to raise the money," said Ruiz. "They were putting up these walls and I did not have near the $2 million." Blocker wrote

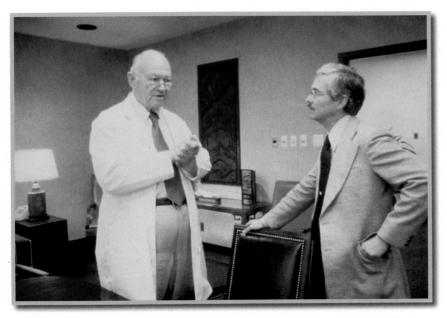

Truman G. Blocker, MD, interim president UT-Health Science Center, Houston and Richard Ruiz, 1977.

many letters to foundations and philanthropists on behalf of Ruiz and the Hermann Eye Center. These letters of endorsement from the legendary and well-respected president of The University of Texas Health Science Center at Houston carried a great deal of credibility and prestige. According to Ruiz, they proved to be the difference between success and failure. "And he never turned me down," said Ruiz. "Not one time."[11]

Blocker's influence and connections proved invaluable. On one occasion, Blocker asked Ruiz if he would come to Galveston and look in on a friend of his, Mary Moody Northen. Northen was chair of the Moody Foundation and the daughter of William L. Moody Jr., patriarch of the powerful Moody family of Galveston. She was suffering from cataracts, but reluctant to seek medical help. Ruiz went with Blocker to the family mansion to meet Northen. Although she insisted that she did not have time for any operation, Blocker convinced her to come to Houston so Ruiz could conduct a thorough examination of her eyes. "Sure

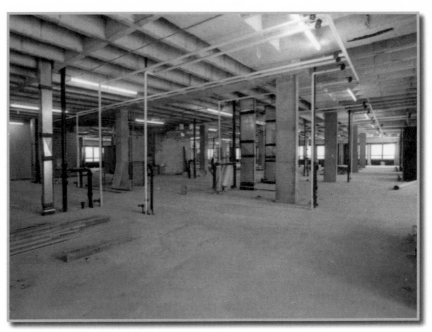

Hermann Eye Center under construction, 1976.

enough, she had real dense cataracts," said Ruiz. "I talked her into doing [the surgery] here at Hermann. However, she would not stay overnight in the hospital, as was customary at the time, so I arranged for her to stay at the Warwick Hotel with an overnight nurse. She got a nice result and they were very appreciative." Ruiz asked if she would be interested in contributing to the Eye Center. To his surprise, the Moody Foundation donated $500,000 to the Hermann Eye Fund. The large donation required Ruiz to change the organizational status of the Eye Fund to comply with government regulations, because as a public charity, no contribution from a single donor could exceed 10 percent of the total dollar amount of donations in a calendar year. It proved to be a beneficial move over the long term, and Ruiz, with legal guidance from two trusted friends, George Hrdlicka, who represented the Hermann Eye Fund, and Randy Gleason, representing Hermann Hospital, was happy to make the changes.[12]

During this time, however, the first signs of discontent began to appear among the doctors of Houston Eye Associates (HEA). Dick Ruiz continued seeing his patients while spending more and more time trying to raise funds for the new Eye Center and supervising the build-out, all with very little involvement from his associates. The ophthalmology practice had grown to the point where Houston Eye Associates occupied the entire eleventh floor of the Hermann Professional Building and expanded into part of the twelfth floor. With their successful, booming practices, some of the doctors were reluctant to embrace fully Ruiz's notion of how the Hermann Eye Center would operate. "My associates were all good people and good doctors who were just interested in their practice," recalled Ruiz. "We had a parting of the ways about exactly what we were going to do with this Eye Center. I could see that we were going down divergent paths and they were more interested in private practice rather than practice plus teaching and research. I got a little bit embittered because I had to do all that fundraising by myself and I did not get any help from anybody over there. I also felt that many of the Houston Eye Associates did not have a sense of loyalty to Hermann Hospital or to The University of Texas Medical School."[13]

Despite this initial fall out, and as construction and fundraising continued during the next several months, Dick Ruiz took a major role in planning the design and layout of the Hermann Eye Center. The goal was to provide complete eye care in one location with a focus on ensuring an efficient flow of patients through the Center. The new Eye Center would offer integrated ophthalmic units in one location, including a glaucoma unit, a photography suite, an orthoptic facility, an electrodiagnostic unit, ultrasonography equipment, a pediatric unit, and a low-vision center. The Hermann Eye Center also included offices for the State Commission for the Blind, the Delta Gamma Counseling Service, an optical shop, and for a time, a pharmacy. There was a separate area to prepare patients for exams and routine contact lens check-ups, eliminating the need to occupy exam rooms for preliminary procedures and improving patient flow. The facility offered two "quick-check" areas that could assist up to six patients, which primarily served to provide examinations for postoperative cataract surgery and for routine glaucoma check-ups.[14]

Another unique component of the Hermann Eye Center was the original artwork Ruiz planned to display throughout the facility. Dick Ruiz always enjoyed art and sculpture, and believed from the beginning of his career that displaying art in the eye clinic would enhance the patients' experience. He wanted to display works of art that could be enjoyed by visually impaired patients as well as by those with good eyesight. Ruiz realized that abstract paintings, particularly larger pieces with bright, vibrant colors and designs, would do this as well as help create a cheerful atmosphere in the Eye Center. Over the years, he collected interesting paintings and, as time passed, found that local artists were willing to loan and even donate pieces for the Eye Center. Thus, the art work brought pleasure for the patients and employees, and gave local artists exposure as well. After a well-known Houston gallery owner and art dealer, Ben DuBose, died of a malignant mela-

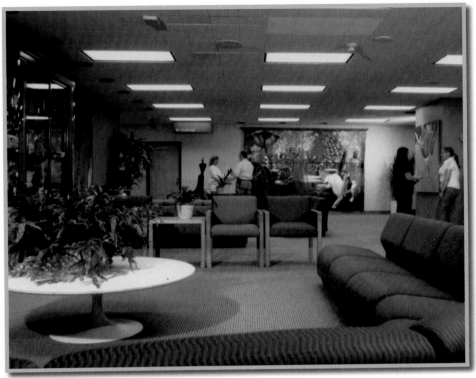

Hermann Eye Center reception area and waiting room.

noma of the eye, Ruiz asked two well-known local artists, David
Adickes and Herb Mears, if they would be interested in donating
paintings to Hermann Eye Center's collection in his memory. Dubose had been very supportive of their work for many years and
they were more than happy to make the donations in memory of
their good friend. Subsequently, works of many other artists have
been donated or acquired for the collection, including those of
Dixon Bennett, Lamar Briggs, David Hickman, Al Kaeppel, Peggy
Oxford, Oris Robertson, and Gonzales Tornero.[15]

  With most of the components in place, the Hermann Eye
Center began seeing patients on a limited basis in October 1977,
with a formal opening a few weeks later, on December 8. But only
Dick Ruiz and Dr. Charles Garcia actually moved into the new
facility. Garcia trained under Ruiz as an ophthalmology resident

at Hermann Hospital, and, in 1973, was in the first graduating class of residents from The University of Texas Medical School at Houston. "I was actually the first person in the Hermann Eye Center seeing patients," Garcia remembered. "I predated Dick by about ten days." Garcia was attracted by Ruiz's idea that a private practice group would be the basis for the department in the medical school. In time, Ruiz envisioned opening satellite offices in the suburbs with the Hermann Eye Center as the hub. "It was a great idea, a super idea, and I was very attracted to that," said Garcia. "He has a tremendous talent for visualizing structures that would be innovative and would be self-sustaining. He, in many ways, was a visionary for how academic ophthalmology would evolve."[16]

Shortly after the Eye Center opened, Sue McRaney joined the program as a social worker sponsored by the Delta Gamma Alumni Association, a volunteer group that worked primarily

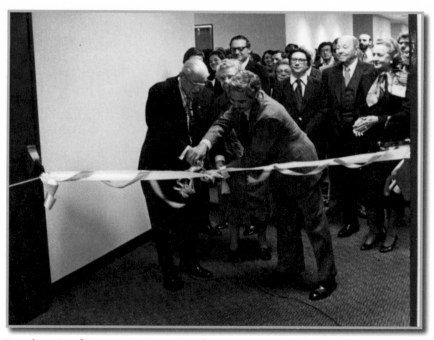

Formal opening of Hermann Eye Center, December 1977.

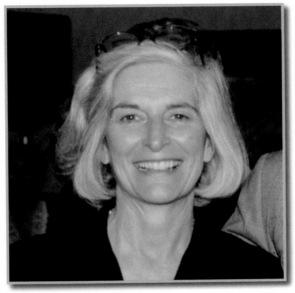

Sue McRaney joined the Eye Center in 1977 as a social worker with the Delta Gamma Alumni Association and became manager of the Eye Clinic in 1983.

with children. Delta Gamma Sorority chapters across the nation provided funds to assist the visually handicapped and the blind. Ruiz planned that the Houston Delta Gamma Foundation for the Visually Handicapped would be an integral part of the Hermann Eye Center, offering professional counseling to patients and also to the parents of visually impaired children. The Delta Gammas provided information about schools and agencies that offered additional services, and also trained volunteers to work in the Eye Center assisting patients and developing follow-up programs for them. Sue McRaney initially started working with blind children who were patients in the Eye Center, but as more patients came through, she found herself working with adults as well. McRaney helped connect people with other social services and worked closely with the Hermann Eye Fund to get financial assistance for those in need. Her interpersonal skills, dedication, and professionalism greatly impressed the staff. Several years later, in 1983, Dr. Ruiz asked McRaney to take on the responsibilities of being the overall manager of the clinic in addition to continuing to provide social services.[17]

With a new facility and several new people joining the Hermann Eye Center, Ruiz decided to launch a new publication, *Views & Visions*, a newsletter about the latest important happenings in the Center that also provided information on recent research and treatments for diseases of the eye. The inaugural issue proclaimed, "The purpose of the Center is to assure that each patient receives optimal care, by a combination of professional expertise with the latest in ophthalmic equipment." The magazine listed several goals for the Eye Center that represented the "ideals of the Director and staff of the Hermann Eye Center" and that also could serve as guidelines for developing future eye centers. The goals included providing the best eye care possible; personalized service for each patient; a referral service for patients with difficult diagnostic and therapeutic problems; and free professional service to indigent patients with serious eye problems. Academic goals included providing a center for teaching ophthalmology by curriculum and by practical experience; providing a dynamic, stimulating milieu for the development of innovative forms of diagnosis and treatment; flexibility to adapt to new developments in treatment methods, equipment and eye care concepts; and facilities for an active research program responsive to the practical needs of ophthalmology. Other goals included providing supplementary services such as patient education, rehabilitation and social counseling; and administrative goals to assure a fiscally responsible organization managed according to sound business principles.[18]

Just prior to the opening of the Hermann Eye Center, Ruiz observed that construction was wrapping up on the new medical school building, but work had not yet begun on refurbishing the Hermann Hospital's main building, the Corbin J. and Wilhelmina C. Robertson Pavilion of Hermann Hospital. Ruiz conveyed his frustration with the delay in a letter to William F. Smith, Executive Director of Hermann Hospital, in August 1977. He expressed

HERMANN EYE CENTER GOALS AND CONCEPTS
A GUIDE TO THE FUTURE

The goals and concepts of Hermann Eye Center represent the ideals of the Director and staff of Hermann Eye Center and serve as guidelines for the development of future centers. These goals are:

• to provide the best eye care possible, including screening, diagnosis and treatment for the full range of visual problems

• to provide personalized service for each patient

• to act as a referral service for patients with difficult diagnostic and therapeutic problems

• to provide free professional service to indigent patients with serious eye problems

• to provide a center for teaching ophthalmology by curriculum and by practical experience

• to provide a dynamic, stimulating milieu for the development of innovative forms of diagnosis and treatment

• to provide a flexible environment capable of responding to future changes in patient flow and new developments in treatment methods, equipment and eye care concepts

• to provide facilities for an active research program responsive to the practical needs of ophthalmology

• to provide ancillary services such as patient education, rehabilitation and social counseling

his concerns about the "general disorganization and lack of efficiency in the Ophthalmology Surgical Service" and that "eye patients are spread all over the Hermann complex." His exhortation to "get started with the construction of the Surgery Suite in the Robertson Pavilion and the renovation of the in-patient rooms" seemed to get lost in the internal affairs of the hospital. Another year would pass before construction on the Robertson Pavilion renovations actually began.[19]

Ruiz's plan for the Hospitalized Eye Patient Unit called for eye patients to be located in one area—on the seventh floor of the Robertson Pavilion—instead of scattered throughout Hermann Hospital, where they received care from staff who also treated other types of patients. If the eye patients were housed in one area, they could be cared for by "a core of personnel" trained to care for ophthalmic patients; the eye patients would receive specialized nursing care from ophthalmic nurses, and the eye surgeons would work with the same staff team for all of their patients. Recognizing that the typical eye patient was not necessarily "sick," Ruiz designed the new facilities to treat both bedridden patients and also those who required very little nursing care and who were completely ambulatory. Therefore, the ambulatory patients could enjoy a degree of freedom and mobility during their hospital stay, at a reduced cost. Other options would be created specifically for eye patients, including a dining area and meeting place where they could enjoy meals outside of their rooms and socialize with visitors and other eye patients. This model would be both patient-friendly and cost effective.[20]

But in the end, this concept of a separate eye surgery suite with its efficient, streamlined service for both inpatients and outpatients did not come to fruition. Engineers discovered structural problems on the seventh floor of the Robertson Pavilion—too much vibration in beams where delicate surgical microscopes were to be mounted—that made the development of an eye surgery suite impossible. Because Ruiz thought that the eye surgery suite would be placed on the seventh floor of the Robertson Pavilion, the opportunity to have a specialized eye surgery suite in the main operating room, which then was under expansion, was no longer possible. Instead, Ruiz and the eye doctors would have to continue using operating rooms on the second floor of the hospital and had lost the opportunity to design specialized surgical rooms in the main operating suite. A day surgery service for all of the hospital's surgical services, utilizing the main operating room, opened on March 6, 1979. This offered better service for the Eye Center's patients. It also reduced patients' costs by an estimated 20–50 percent. Instead of checking in at the hospital's emergency room and having surgery in one of the nearby operating rooms, eye surgery patients now checked in at the nurses' station in the Eye Unit. Patients no longer endured the uncertainties and delays caused by the "chaotic and abnormal routine" of the emergency room. They could remain in their street clothes for their surgery, and had the comfort of knowing that family or friends were nearby. Although eye surgeons used the day surgery suite, it was not equipped for all types of eye surgery. But for patients who suffered from retinal tears, diabetic retinopathy, Coates' disease, sickle cell retinopathy, acute glaucoma, and cataracts that could be treated with outpatient surgery, it was a tremendous relief and convenience.[21]

Despite the cancellation of the planned facilities in the Robertson Pavilion, by 1980, the new Hermann Eye Center was seeing over 120 patients per day on average, and gaining recognition as a leader in providing high quality eye care to patients. Visitors from Cornell University, the University of Oregon, and St. Louis University in Missouri, all considering the creation of their own eye centers, came to Hermann Eye Center to see how it operated. Texas Tech University sent architects to glean ideas from the Hermann Eye Center. Dr. Julio Bueso, of the Instituto Ramon y Cajal in Madrid, came all the way from Spain to spend a month observing the Eye Center. Local television stations also became interested, and a Canadian television company included the Eye Center as part of its documentary on The University of Texas Medical School and Hermann Hospital.[22]

While the Hermann Eye Center was becoming known as a center of excellence in eye care, behind the scenes an emerging difference of opinion on the role of Houston Eye Associates and their relationship with the Hermann Eye Center was developing into a major split among the partners. As is the case in many partnerships, success often brings conflicting strategic visions for how the enterprise should continue to operate. As already mentioned, the first signs of disagreement over the future of Houston Eye Associates (HEA) occurred a few years earlier when most of the associates failed to embrace Dick Ruiz's idea for the Eye Center or to assist in his fundraising campaign for the seventh floor of the Jones Pavilion. Houston Eye Associates had its offices across the street from the hospital and the new medical school, and several of the partners did not see much benefit in moving to what they viewed as a more congested area of the Texas Medical Center (TMC). Although many of the doctors enjoyed teaching and working with the medical students, for them it was not the primary focus in their professional lives. They had gone to medical school and taken specialized training in ophthalmology mainly to have a private practice, see patients, and to earn a good living. They shared neither Dick Ruiz's deep enthusiasm nor his dedication to teaching, an endeavor that required personal sacrifice and significant blocks of time if they were to fulfill his model for the Eye Center. Charles Russo, the first to join Ruiz as a partner in 1967, recalled that "Dick left the Hermann Professional Building and did his entire practice over there. Some of us would go over from time to time and see patients, and then that began to dwindle down. Dick had the idea of being totally obligated to the Hermann Eye Center. Well, some of us didn't share that idea."[23]

Indeed, after the Hermann Eye Center opened, most of the physicians from Houston Eye Associates saw some patients, mostly new patients referred from the hospital, in the new facility, but they did not actually move into it. They continued seeing their regular patients across the street in the Hermann Professional Building. As their practices grew and new associates came on board, they decided that they needed a new, more expansive workplace. They wanted an office in a building that they owned and in which they did not have to pay rent; one that they felt would be more accessible for patients to visit, with fewer parking problems and less traffic congestion than the area around the Hermann Eye Center and the Hermann Professional Building.[24]

Administratively, they viewed the Hermann Eye Center, which was where Dick Ruiz now worked exclusively, as a cost center for the main office in the Hermann Professional Building. By contrast, Ruiz viewed it as the hub for what one day would be multiple "spokes" leading to satellite eye clinics around the city. In his mind, patients would have standard ophthalmic needs treated at the satellite locations and would come to the main Hermann Eye Center in the TMC for specialized diagnosis and treatments. This fundamental difference of opinion regarding the relationship of Houston Eye Associates and the Hermann Eye Center continued to develop, but both Ruiz and his partners tried to make the best of the situation.

After several months of searching for a location, Houston Eye Associates purchased land for their new building from Dr. John P. McGovern, a well-known Houston allergist and philanthropist. The site was opposite the Hermann Hospital Outpatient Surgery Center on Gramercy Street, a block from Holcombe Boulevard, and about ten minutes from the Texas Medical Center.[25] In 1984, they broke ground for a new three-story building and moved into it the following year. By this time, Dick Ruiz focused primarily on the Hermann Eye Center and on his duties as chair of the department of ophthalmology in the medical school. He had little to do administratively with HEA. Several of the original partners from Houston Eye Associates continued to teach in the medical school and to see patients at the Hermann Eye Center. However, when patients began their eye care at the Hermann Eye Center, once they learned that they could see the same ophthalmologist at the new building, with its ample surface parking away from the congestion of the Texas Medical Center, they usually chose the Gramercy Street location for their follow-up visits. This patient drain meant that the Hermann Eye Center struggled to build up a stable patient base while HEA pushed to build up patient flow at the Gramercy Street office in order to pay for the new building. Consequently, the two offices found themselves in competition for the same patients, which resulted in a financially troublesome effect on the Hermann Eye Center.

Additionally, Ruiz was devoted to building the department of ophthalmology in the medical school. As department chair, he was responsible for hiring faculty and running the academic component of the Eye Center. Demands on HEA doctors to devote more time to the medical school, time for which they did not receive compensation, created more anxiety within the group as the concurrent needs of their own growing private practices increased. "I think they felt like it was an okay idea, but I don't think they were able to grasp the significance and long-term benefits of the association with the university and the hospital," Ruiz later observed. "Most were, to some degree, at least in those early days, pretty interested in teaching. But most of them lost that interest. As they got busier and busier in practice, it was a matter of either seeing their own patients and being paid for it or teaching somebody and not being paid for it." In addition, Ruiz was very loyal to Hermann Hospital and had pledged to fully support that institution during his negotiations to create the Eye Center. But now, he felt that most of his partners in Houston Eye Associates shared neither his loyalty to Hermann nor his commitment to UT. "The individual Houston Eye Associates were happy to display an academic title from UT and for the group to be considered synonymous with the faculty of the department of ophthalmology, which lent an aura of excellence and prestige," said Ruiz. "But only a few were willing to help carry out the mission of Hermann Hospital and the medical school. The premise on which the group was founded was forgotten, and so, we drifted further and further apart."[26]

After fifteen increasingly awkward years of trying to accommodate these disparate views within Houston Eye Associates, Dick Ruiz reached the painful conclusion that their association no longer made sense. The Gramercy Street office and the Hermann Eye Center were operating at cross purposes administratively and economically, and under irreconcilable differences philosophically. Ruiz did not like being just a cost center in Houston Eye Associates' business structure, and worried that in time, when he stepped down as department chair in the medical school, his successor would be in an impossible situation: "one little cog in a big corporate wheel, with no control over anything, including medical records, billing, and collections." He decided that in the best interests of the ophthalmology department, the medical school, and the hospital, his only alternative was to leave HEA. Charles Garcia, who continued to see patients in the Hermann Eye Center, later observed that the breakup "occurred for the same reason all of these splits occurred: there came a divergence of [opinion about] the appropriate vision for the organization. Neither one was right nor wrong; they just grew apart. The people at HEA were more interested in the new building and maintaining a certain level of independence from the school. And Dick was more interested in having the [eye center] and school be the hub, and not a spoke."[27]

Ruiz informed Houston Eye Associates of his decision and began to work out the details with Dr. Jeffrey Lanier, who was president of the group at that time. Lanier later recalled, "In 1992, it was determined that we really needed to split for the benefit of both. ... they needed to build a department of ophthalmologists that were exclusively there at the Hermann Eye Center to teach the residents and be with the residents." Negotiating the split took nearly two years. Ruiz asked for his patient records, which technically belonged to HEA. Financial issues also had to be negotiated in the divestment agreement. In many ways, the breakup was much like a divorce, and while it was not pleasant, it could have turned into a very ugly situation. "Dr. Ruiz and I worked all this out about the separation," said Lanier. "It is a very cordial, agreed-upon separation and worked very well." Some of Ruiz's original partners attempted to dissuade him, but in the end, they agreed to the split. It was a difficult situation, but, as Ruiz recalled later, "they were gentlemanly about it."[28]

The breakup of Houston Eye Associates and the Hermann Eye Center was a bitter disappointment for doctors in both camps. Years later, Dr. Charles Russo, the first to join with Ruiz in 1967, recalled, "Certainly, there were hard feelings. There sure were. But it wasn't anything that anybody couldn't handle; let's put it that way. As time has worked it out, he has been very successful over there; we have been very successful over here." Dr. Malcolm Mazow offered a similar perspective, observing, "The different philosophies are the things that made the ultimate split, and there were some hard feelings on both sides. But that is how the split came about, and, you know, the divorce happens and you go on and go forward. It is as simple as that."

It is tempting to speculate on what might have been had the group found a way to bring their divergent views into one strategic vision. Instead of being in competition for patients, the suburban offices that later comprised Houston Eye Associates might have been the "satellites" that Dick Ruiz envisioned as radiating out from the Hermann Eye Center's "hub" in the Texas Medical Center. And the affiliation with The University of Texas Medical School and the Hermann Eye Center would have brought additional prestige and further enhanced the reputation of Houston Eye Associates. "So, had [things] worked out like I thought they could, we would have been way ahead of the game, because we had a huge private practice," said Ruiz. And Malcolm Mazow observed that "the divorce didn't need to occur, [if] more level heads [had looked] forward to what would have been better for everybody concerned."[29]

Dick Ruiz now found himself in a very challenging position. His dream for a comprehensive, world-class eye center had not died, but it definitely was in jeopardy. The patient base that remained was comprised of Ruiz's private practice and Hermann Hospital's indigent clinic patients. But now, he would have to recruit new doctors to join the practice and recruit new faculty as a foundation to build the department of ophthalmology into the kind of eye center he envisioned years before. A man of deep conviction, Ruiz was not afraid of challenge or of hard work. He was, however, approaching the age at which many choose to retire and yet embarking on a task many younger men would refuse to undertake. But for Dick Ruiz, there was no other choice.

Thirty years after opening his ophthalmology practice in Houston, Dick Ruiz found himself facing one of the major challenges of his professional life. He was dedicated to medicine, to his patients, and to fulfilling his dream of not merely creating but fully developing an exceptional eye center at Hermann Hospital and The University of Texas Medical School. The milestones in his early career—developing a successful ophthalmology practice, his appointment as chief of ophthalmology at Hermann Hospital, and his successful efforts to raise the professional standards in the hospital's ophthalmology training programs—might have been fulfilling on their own. But when The University of Texas announced that it would build a medical school in Houston with Hermann Hospital as its primary teaching hospital, Ruiz saw a once-in-a-lifetime opportunity to create something that truly was exceptional. The concept of bringing together a medical school, teaching hospital, and a private ophthalmology practice into one unit that offered the best in patient care, education, and research was something that, if it succeeded, could create a new model for medical education. The field of ophthalmology already was known as a leader in raising professional standards in medicine. The Hermann Eye Center, as envisioned by Dick Ruiz, held the potential to set a new standard of excellence in ophthalmic education.

Although the new medical school brought great opportunities to the Texas Medical Center, it also created many new and unexpected problems. Administrators at both Hermann Hospital and The University of Texas Medical School had to develop procedures and protocols to govern how the two institutions would interact. This affiliation strained the hospital's financial resources as it struggled to complete the renovations required to meet the needs of the school. And, disillusionment over the nature of the relationship between the hospital's medical staff and the medical school led many of Hermann's doctors to abandon the hospital. Many of Hermann's private practice physicians found the standards of the medical school intolerable. Further, many felt the requirement to submit to the authority of the school's departmental chairs as service chiefs in the hospital—with its potential loss of autonomy over decisions regarding patient care—to be unacceptable.

In a similar way, such perceived conflicts in loyalty placed a strain on Houston Eye Associates, the doctors on whom Dick Ruiz counted to support the Hermann Eye Center and Hermann Hospital and to teach in the department of ophthalmology of the medical school. It was one thing for the doctors of Houston Eye Associates to work with residents and interns on a voluntary basis in the training program at Hermann Hospital. But meeting the more formal demands of serving as faculty in the medical school and fully participating in the Hermann Eye Center required a different level of commitment. The doctors enjoyed the status conferred by their part-time academic appointments but received no financial compensation from the medical school. Thus, although Ruiz and his partners had much in common, including their devotion to excellence in ophthalmology and patient care, they shared neither the same passion for academe nor the same enthusiasm for the concept of the Eye Center. The corporate goals of Houston Eye Associates simply did not mesh with the academic goals that were at the heart of his model for the Eye Center.

The split was a major setback for Dick Ruiz and the Hermann

Eye Center. However, Ruiz had a large private practice in addition to the flow of new patients who were automatically referred because of the Hermann Eye Center's affiliation with Hermann Hospital and The University of Texas Medical School. Thus, he quickly cultivated a new, expanding base of ophthalmology patients. The challenge now was to reinvent the Eye Center using the lessons of the past fifteen years, to recruit new faculty with a firm commitment to academics as well as private practice, and to provide a level of treatment for the patients that made them want to return, in spite of the inconveniences of the Texas Medical Center. What had to be done, then, was clear. But, the health care world in which the Hermann Eye Center was born had entered a new era of change. Within a few years, Ruiz and the Eye Center would encounter that new reality head-on—with surprising ramifications.

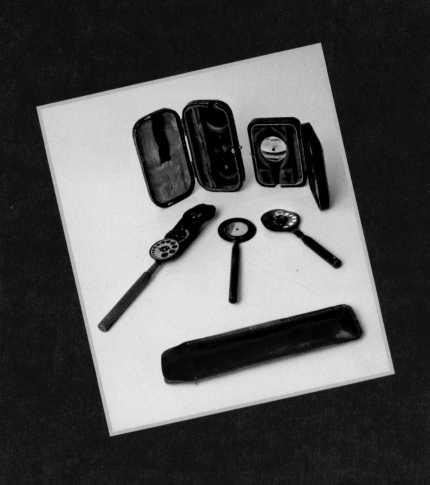

CHAPTER FIVE

Growing Stronger through Times of Change

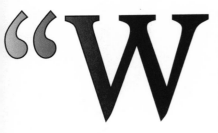ELL, IT WAS LIKE starting from square one again," said Dick Ruiz. "It was fairly slow going ... you can't just start all at once."[1] In the fall of 1993, after the split from Houston Eye Associates (HEA), Ruiz began the process of rebuilding the clinical faculty to serve patients in the eye clinic and teach medical students, residents, and fellows. It also was necessary to create a new business entity to operate the clinical practice. Ruiz, together with his administrative team of Sue McRaney, Joseph Leopold, Glen Knotts, and the Hermann Eye Center staff, faced an enormous challenge, but they never lost confidence in their ability to succeed. With a lot of fortitude and hard work Ruiz and his team continued to provide the high level of patient care and teaching for which the Eye Center had become known. And, in the midst of this rebuilding process, Ruiz was about to score something of a coup by bringing one of the Health Science Center's key research groups back into the ophthalmology department, a move that brought new opportunities to both groups and enhanced the reputation of the department.[2]

While all of this moved forward, the administrative services, which previously had been provided by Houston Eye Associ-

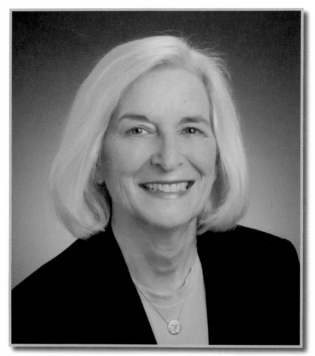

Sue McRaney, Manager, Cizik Eye Clinic

ates, had to be completely restructured. Before the breakup with Houston Eye Associates, the corporate office on Gramercy Street handled all of the administrative work for the ophthalmology practice. As Ruiz began to take over full responsibility for administering the Hermann Eye Center, several key people stayed with him. Sue McRaney, who originally started at the Eye Center as a part-time social worker, now took broader responsibilities in her role as clinic manager. "She was obviously a very capable person, an indefatigable worker, and a leader," said Ruiz. "Earlier, I talked her into going full-time and being the manager of the Eye Center as well as continuing the social work. She has been here ever since, doing whatever we needed for the Eye Center. Over the years she built a great team, played a key role in fundraising, and has done a magnificent job for us." Another key person who chose to remain with Ruiz was the accountant, Joseph Leopold.

After a career in which he rose to vice president of a Louisiana-based wholesale company, Leopold retired and then migrated to Houston where, in 1988, he decided to go back to work as a book-keeper and accountant with Houston Eye Associates. In March 1993, he was moved from the Associates' Gramercy Street office and assigned to work at the Hermann Eye Center. By September, as the separation became final, Leopold determined that he preferred to continue working with Dick Ruiz. "I wanted very much to stay with Dr. Ruiz," Leopold recalled later. "I met with him and asked him if I could have a job in his new outfit. He told me he was not sure where the money was coming from and I said, 'If you are going to risk it at your age, I sure can, too.' And so, we did." McRaney and Leopold proved to be just as dedicated as Ruiz to rebuilding the Eye Center, and over the years assembled an administrative staff that was remarkable for its stability, professionalism, and loyalty. "Those two people have been absolutely critical in the development of the administrative side of it," Ruiz acknowledged. "And then, we've got many other people under them who just turned out to be super."[3]

In addition to McRaney and Leopold, Glenn R. Knotts, PhD, the executive director of the Hermann Eye Fund, also chose to stay with Ruiz. Knotts had a distinguished career prior to joining the Hermann Eye Center in 1989. He had served in numerous academic and administrative positions, including appointments at the American Medical Association, American School Health Association, Kent State University, The University of Texas M.

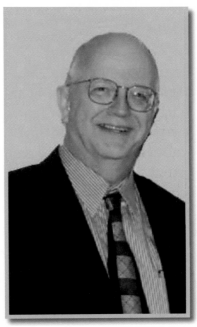

Joseph Leopold, CFO, 1992-2010.

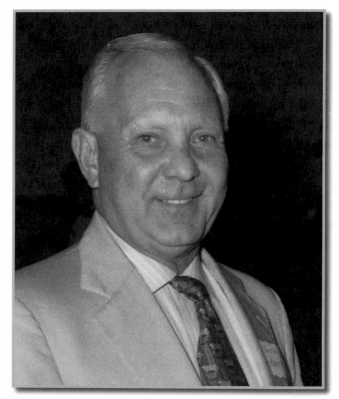

Glenn R. Knotts, PhD, Executive Director, Hermann Eye Fund, 1989-2003.

D. Anderson Cancer Center, the UT Health Science Center, and the John P. McGovern Foundation. Knotts was well acquainted with the major players in Houston's philanthropic community and proved to be particularly charming and adept in one-on-one situations. A stylish dresser with impeccable manners and a genuine thoughtfulness of others, Knotts became an endearing figure in the Hermann Eye Center. Dick Ruiz later said that Knotts was "my good friend, counselor, colleague, fundraiser, coworker, and companion in a cause which we both strongly believed in and truly loved—the Hermann Eye Center and the Department of Ophthalmology and Visual Science."[4]

Under the terms of the separation agreement between Ruiz and Houston Eye Associates, none of the HEA physicians were permitted to see patients at the Hermann Eye Center. But three key people—two eye doctors and a clinical researcher—did remain with Ruiz and together these four formed the nucleus around which a new team of physician/academicians developed. Charles A. Garcia, MD, continued to see patients part-time at the Hermann Eye Center while developing his practice at St. Joseph's and elsewhere. In December 1992, Ruiz recommended Garcia for the Bernice Weingarten Distinguished Professorship in Ophthalmology at The University of Texas Medical School. Already highly regarded for his research, teaching, and patient care, Garcia continued his part-time affiliation with the Hermann Eye Center throughout his career.[5]

Thomas C. Prager, PhD, a clinical researcher, also stayed with Ruiz. Prager received his BA, MS, and PhD degrees from Tulane University. He had been with the Hermann Eye Center since taking a fellowship in the ophthalmology department in ultrasound and electrophysiology with Dr. Garcia in 1979. Prager became a clinical professor in the Department of Ophthalmology and Visual Science and developed a highly regarded electrodiagnostic unit and an ultrasound laboratory of international renown. He also earned a master's degree in public health from The University of Texas School of Public Health while working full-time at the Hermann Eye Center. "Dr. Charlie Garcia recruited me to do a fellowship," said Prager. "I met him at an eye meeting. My areas of interest were pretty much rarified niches: ultrasonog-

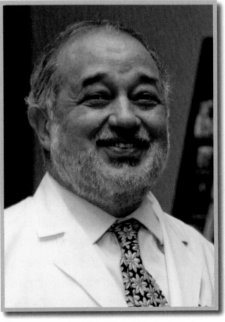

Charles A. Garcia, MD, Clinical Professor and Bernice Weingarten Chair.

raphy and electrophysiology in ophthalmology. Nobody else really wanted to do it."[6]

The third doctor in the group was no stranger to Hermann Hospital or the Hermann Eye Center. In fact, Judianne Kellaway, MD, was born in Hermann Hospital. Her father, Peter Kellaway, PhD, was an internationally known neurophysiologist at Baylor College of Medicine who pioneered the development of electroencephalography (EEG). During her high school years, Judianne Kellaway worked summers and weekends helping her father, often in the basement of Hermann Hospital doing EEGs. After earning both bachelor's and master's degrees in education, Kellaway enjoyed a successful career as a kindergarten teacher. Later, she decided to pursue a medical degree and work in pediatrics. But attending a lab session that exposed students to the inner workings of the human eye hooked Kellaway on ophthalmology. Ultimately, she completed her ophthalmology residency with Dr. Ruiz in 1992. "I was here and I just stayed here," she recalled. "I liked the academic setting, and I had a background in education.... I just wanted to be here and continue to contribute to the patient care that we were able to give, and to teaching the residents and medical students."[7]

With this cadre of key people in place, one of Ruiz's first tasks was to create a new corporate structure for the clinical practice. During the fall of 1993, he established the Hermann/University Eye Associates (later referred to as University Eye Associates or UEA), a not-for-profit corporation. "I thought that was a better way to go, since it was my intention to align clearly the goals of the Hermann Eye Center so that they would be inextricably wedded to the hospital and the Medical School," said Ruiz. "I thought that a not-for-profit entity would interface better with those two not-for-profit institutions and, looking back, it has worked out well."[8]

Ruiz announced the formation of University Eye Associates in the Eye Center's *Views & Visions* publication several months later during the fall of 1994. The article emphasized that all of the doctors were "dedicated faculty members of the Department of Ophthalmology and Visual Science at The University of Texas Medical School." The brief statement noted that Ruiz originally founded Houston Eye Associates to combine private practice with the teaching and research goals of the Department of Ophthalmology. But as the original group varied from those guidelines, Ruiz determined that it was "appropriate to leave the old corporation and establish a new group truly dedicated to teaching and research as well as patient care." With the new corporate structure in place, McRaney and Leopold could develop the administrative systems the Eye Center needed.

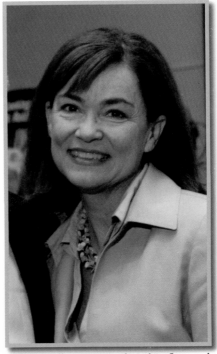

Judianne Kellaway, MD., Clinical Professor and Stephen Lasher Professor.

New patients mainly came by way of the emergency room at Hermann Hospital and through referrals from faculty at the medical school. Ruiz already had a fine reputation and large patient base, and the Eye Center continued to attract new patients by virtue of its expertise and research. "We had a good stream of patients and income right from the beginning," Ruiz remembered. "And we never went in the red after separating from Houston Eye Associates."[9]

Although the newly constituted University Eye Associates kept Dick Ruiz extremely busy, he was always looking for opportunities to enhance the Eye Center. Sometime during 1991 or early 1992, he discovered that officials at The University of Texas Health Science Center wanted to reorganize the Graduate School of Biomedical Sciences by amalgamating its research centers, including the Sensory Sciences Center (SSC), into the medical school. Harry Sperling, PhD, first established the Sensory Sciences Center in 1967. Sperling, a highly regarded scientist, had done extensive research in color vision for the U.S. Navy and wrote a doctoral dissertation on spectral sensitivity of the eye. Prior to his move to Houston, he spent nine years at Honeywell Inc., where he rose from senior scientist to manager of life sciences. With this diverse background, in 1967, Sperling was appointed professor in the UT Graduate School of Biomedical Sciences. During the next twenty-eight years, Sperling developed a group of scientists who conducted research and taught in The University of Texas Graduate School of Biomedical Sciences, and later, in the medical school. They conducted research in various human sensory processes with an emphasis on the brain's processing of sensory information, which included the retina, color processing, vision, taste, and smell. The SSC had been part of the Graduate School of Biomedical Sciences from its founding until 1978, when, under the urging of acting president Truman G. Blocker, the SSC moved to the ophthalmology department.[10] Dick Ruiz later recalled that during a meeting one afternoon, Blocker had turned toward him and said, "Hey Ruiz, why don't you take that SSC group and put them in ophthalmology?" Blocker apparently thought that because of all the vision research conducted by the scientists of the SSC, its natural home was in ophthalmology. A startled Ruiz replied, "Well, if we could get an adequate budget to support them, I would be delighted!" But just five years later, in 1983, Ernst Knobil, dean of the medical school, was faced with the task of recruiting five new department chairpersons, and asked that because of space needs, the SSC be moved back to the Graduate School of Biomedical Sciences. Thus, because the SSC previously had been part of the Department of Ophthalmology, and because so much of their research dealt with the visual system, many of the scientists had secondary appointments in ophthalmology and were well-known to the chair of the department, Dick Ruiz.[11]

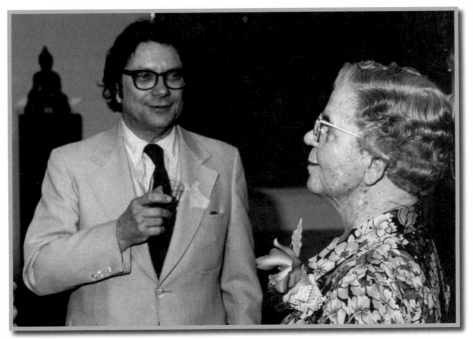

Harry Sperling, PhD, founding director, UT-Sensory Sciences Center, 1967-1995, with Elizabeth Morford, a patient and benefactor of the Hermann Eye Center.

When the UT administration decided to move these researchers to the medical school, some there assumed that the Sensory Sciences Center would fit best in the Department of Neurobiology and Anatomy. But Ruiz believed that with so much of their research centered on the eye and visual system, the obvious and natural new home for the majority of the scientists should be in ophthalmology. The sterling reputations of the SSC scientists and the high level of research they conducted would bring new prestige to the department, providing a basic science research component in addition to the clinical research conducted in the Hermann Eye Center. A merger with ophthalmology would transform the department and elevate it to a fully academic unit of the medical school, bringing new possibilities to win lucrative grants to fund research and an opportunity to help UT maintain the research laboratories with accompanying indirect costs. Along with those grants came enhanced opportunity to continue attracting the best and brightest scientists, residents, and medical students. With so much at stake in terms of prestige, state-funded salaries, and potential grant funding, the Department of Neurobiology and Anatomy would not easily acquiesce.

As Dick Ruiz recalled, John H. "Jack" Byrne, PhD, chair of neurobiology and anatomy, argued that the SSC belonged in his department, that he could attract grant funding from Research to Prevent Blindness as well as from the National Institutes of Health, and that since Ruiz was classified only at half-time as ophthalmology chair, he (Byrne) would be better able to administer the SSC. Byrne's position meant that Ruiz had to initiate a major campaign on behalf of the Department of Ophthalmology to bring the vision researchers in the Sensory Sciences Center back into the fold. Ruiz argued that the SSC would flourish if it were part of ophthalmology, and pointed out that Research to Prevent Blindness only offered grants to ophthalmology departments, a statement that later proved to be true. Ultimately, Ruiz and Byrne presented these arguments before a large committee (composed primarily of PhD full-time faculty, a few MDs, and lay people) formed by Dean John C. Ribble to hear the arguments and make a recommendation.

From about mid-1992 to mid-1994, as Ruiz was busy disengaging from Houston Eye Associates, he continued to pursue every avenue to bring the vision researchers of the SSC into the ophthalmology department. After discussing the situation with Dr. Ruiz, Professor Dianna A. Redburn, PhD, a talented and respected researcher in the Department of Neurobiology and Anatomy, formally requested that her primary appointment in the medical school be changed to ophthalmology. Although her transfer to ophthalmology was approved, her state-funded salary line was not moved with her and remained in neurobiology and anatomy. Ruiz later nominated Redburn for the prestigious Jules and Doris Stein Professorship, funded by Research to Prevent Blindness, Inc., of New York, for which she easily won approval. She also had been appointed the titular head of the SSC upon the retirement of Harry Sperling as director. Diana Redburn's impeccable scientific credentials, energy, and organizational skills proved to be crucial during the next few months.[12]

As the time came for the SSC to be dissolved, two of the scientists who were not involved in vision research were placed in the Department of Neurobiology and Anatomy. The five scientists in the group who were doing vision research chose to join ophthalmology. Ruiz had told them that if they clearly expressed their desire to join the ophthalmology department, he was confident that the medical school would honor their request. As Dr. Stephen C. Massey, one of the SSC scientists, remembered later, "We joined the ophthalmology department because a number of people in the Sensory Sciences Center worked specifically on retina and, of course, that seemed appropriate for an ophthalmology depart-

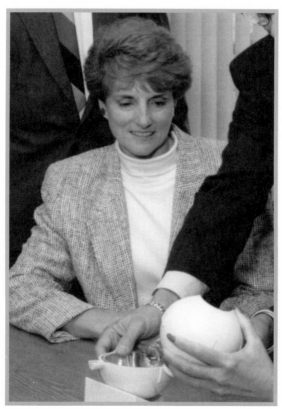

Dianna Redburn, PhD, Professor, UT Medical School, Houston.

ment. And we were welcomed here with open arms." The SSC's department administrator, Ms. Fredi Bleeker (later Fredi Bleeker Franks), at first appeared destined to be placed in neurobiology and anatomy. But Ruiz saw the need for an experienced basic science administrator, now that the SSC's vision researchers had moved back to the Department of Ophthalmology. He told her the same thing he had told the scientists—to insist that she wanted to move to ophthalmology—and in the end, they prevailed. Bleeker had a broad background in office management, clinic management, and personnel management, both in the private sector and at The University of Texas Medical School. She joined the staff of the Sensory Sciences Center as department administrator in 1993, which at the time was part of the Graduate School of Biomedical Sciences. When Jeannie McLemore, the ophthalmology department's chief business administrator, retired in 1997, Ruiz offered the job to Bleeker, thus combining the two administrative functions into one position, director of management operations. With the merger completed, the SSC became known as the Basic Science Group of the Department of Ophthalmology. Ruiz felt it was appropriate to change the name of the department to better represent its increased academic scope. He suggested that it be named the Department of Ophthalmology and Visual Science (DOVS).[13]

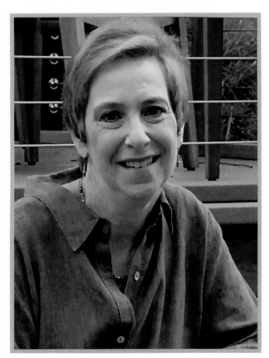

Fredi Bleeker Franks, Director of Management Operations, UT-Department of Ophthalmology.

As this transpired, several scientists in the department, led by Drs. Ruiz, Redburn, and Massey, began thinking about how to apply for additional grant funding in the form of a National Eye Institute (NEI) Vision Core Grant. These prestigious grants were difficult to acquire and, at the time, provided more than $1 million for research. One key way to attract positive attention to a grant proposal was to show that the funds would support a broad group of scientists, as in a research cluster or center, and that the receiving institution also supported the research endeavor. As Steve Massey later recalled, "I don't know who came up with the idea; they called it a consortium. I think somebody must have figured out . . . that actually, there was a lot of vision research here at UT, and if we would just get together as a group, then we would be eligible for this [funding] mechanism." In 1993, Dianna Redburn approached Ruiz with the idea of bringing together all thirty-five researchers from The University of Texas at Houston Health Science Center's Department of Ophthalmology, Department of Neurobiology and Anatomy of the Medical School; the School of Public Health; the Dental Branch; and the Graduate School of Biomedical Sciences in a concerted effort to acquire a Vision Core Grant. Ruiz later said that it was Dianna Redburn who came up with the idea of calling the group a "consortium." The new Vision Research Consortium would be centered and administered through the Department of Ophthalmology and Visual Science, where Dianna A. Redburn, PhD, a full professor, was named director. Redburn also continued as adjunct professor in the Department of Neurobiology and Anatomy, and as the medical school's assistant dean for research training.

The Vision Research Consortium brought together scientists of diverse backgrounds from four of the six UT Health Science Center schools, all of whom were conducting vision research. This created the opportunity to have a research group that could form the vanguard of national and even international visual science research. Additionally, the opportunities for collaborative projects and shared use of expensive equipment made it possible to justify the acquisition of highly advanced instruments that individual researchers simply could not afford to purchase. For Dick Ruiz, Clinical Professor and Chair of the Department of Ophthalmology and Visual Science, bringing the Basic Science Group into the department and forming the Vision Research Consortium meant that there now was the real potential for the department to achieve the exemplary status in vision research that had been one of his original goals in creating the Hermann Eye Center. "The concept of bringing all the talent together for a team approach to visual science within the Health Science Center represents to me what the university should be about," said Ruiz.[14]

One of the first projects the consortium undertook was to obtain a confocal microscope, an expensive piece of equipment that could be used by all members of the group. Although confocal microscopy had been around since the late 1950s, recent developments in the use of lasers and in computer technology had greatly improved their utility. Confocal microscopes used a process called optical sectioning to acquire detailed images of complex specimens. With the use of lasers and computer technology, the confocal microscope produced high-resolution planar (two-dimensional) images of biological structures, and from them created highly detailed three-dimensional images. The ability to see these detailed, microscopic images opened an entirely new world in vision research. Steve Massey took a leadership role in developing possible uses of the microscope by members of the consortium. He quickly saw the value and utility of this new technology. But at a cost of approximately $200,000, the equipment was much too expensive for a single lab to purchase. The Vision Research Consortium, however, with its group of research scientists from several different labs, could make use of this advanced technology in a collaborative, cost-effective manner. Dianna Redburn suggested that the university provide funds for the purchase of a confocal microscope as "seed money" that would help in the quest to receive a National Eye Institute Vision Core Grant. The university tentatively approved funding, provided that the consor-

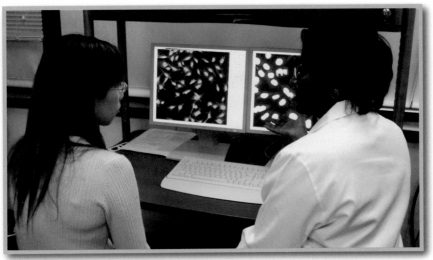

Above, *Researchers view enhanced images from-Confocal Microscope.* Right, *Confocal Microscope.*

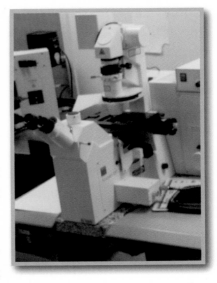

tium received the grant. The confocal microscope demonstrated the institution's support and was seen by many as the jewel in the application. "So, that is how it started," said Steve Massey. "Dianna Redburn wrote that first application and lo and behold, it was funded."[15]

In June 1993, the Vision Research Consortium formally submitted its Vision Core Grant application to the National Eye Institute. Nearly nine months later, on March 1, 1994, the NEI announced that it was awarding a five-year Vision Core Grant of approximately $1,092,000 to The University of Texas at Houston Health Science Center. The core grant, given specifically to the Vision Research Consortium, was to be administered with Dr. Dianna Redburn of the Department of Ophthalmology and Visual Science as the principal investigator. The grant enabled the group's scientists to conduct research in a number of areas including glaucoma, retinal aging, and other primary causes of blindness. The university pledged to install support facilities, provide new analytical computer software, and assemble a biostatistics program connecting research findings with public health data. The confocal microscope was the centerpiece of the planned research program, and the university's willingness to purchase the expensive instrument was considered one of the keys that led the National Eye Institute to award this grant to the Consortium.[16]

These culminating events of 1994 greatly enhanced the reputation of the Department of Ophthalmology and Visual Science. The addition of the Basic Science Group, the formation of the Vision Research Consortium, and the announcement of the Vision Core Grant from the National Eye Institute also raised the profile of the UT–Houston Medical School and of The University of Texas Health Science Center. The Department of Ophthalmology and Visual Science now had the potential to achieve a level of excellence that could draw more funding for research while attracting the most highly qualified faculty and students to the medical school. Ruiz's model for a world-class eye center was coming to fruition at last in the way he first envisioned. Just one year earlier, the prospects for the future of the Hermann Eye Center had been less than promising. Ruiz was determined, however, and he had a dedicated team with which to rebuild. During this difficult time, Hermann Hospital appointed Dr. Ruiz as chief of staff for 1993–94. Although it was not apparent at the time, this honor marked a symbolic turning point for Ruiz and for the Hermann Eye Center at the beginning of a new era of incredibly hard work and enormous success. The momentum carried over into the next few years as Ruiz increased the clinical staff with the addition of several new physicians whose specific areas of expertise made the Hermann Eye Center a place where patients could be treated in one location by a diverse group of leading eye subspecialists.

In 1996, Dianna Redburn left the department for personal reasons—to be near her soon-to-be-husband—and moved to the University of Tennessee Health Science Center at Memphis, where she was appointed professor of ophthalmology and director of research.[17] The loss of the director of basic science research and principal investigator of the Vision Core Grant left a huge void in the department. By this time, Ruiz had had ten years to observe and become acquainted with Steve Massey. Massey, who earned a PhD at London University, had been one of the scientists in the Sensory Science Center and had held an appointment on the UT–Houston faculty since 1985, first in the Graduate School of Biomedical Sciences and later the Medical School. He was a highly regarded scientist known internationally for his research in the anatomy of the retina and how drugs affect retinal function. There was no question of his scientific abilities, but in addition, Ruiz saw that Massey was an able manager and logical thinker with excellent interpersonal skills. Ruiz was delighted when Massey agreed to take on the responsibility as director of basic science and principal investigator of the Vision Core Grant. In 1996, Ruiz appointed Stephen C. Massey to take Redburn's place as director of basic research and as full professor in the Depart-

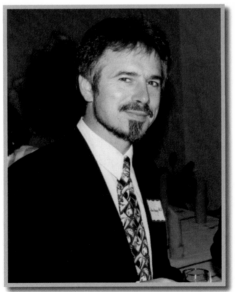

Stephen C. Massey, PhD, Director of Basic Science Research, Professor, and Elizabeth Morford Chair.

ment of Ophthalmology and Visual Science. Ruiz's confidence proved to be well founded; the Basic Science Group continued to thrive under Massey's leadership.[18]

The Department of Ophthalmology and Visual Science continued to attract new funding, enhancing its reputation as a center of excellence in vision research. In 1996, one of the department's scientists, Dr. Stephen L. Mills, received a Dolly Green Scholars Award in the amount of $60,000 from Research to Prevent Blindness (RPB). The $60,000 award provided funding for Mills's research into the causes, treatment, and prevention of blinding diseases. The Dolly Green Scholars Award was part of a special RPB program created "to support outstanding young scientists who are conducting research of unusual significance and promise." In April 1996, Dick Ruiz received special recognition when the Harris County Medical Society's Museum of Health and Medical Science dedicated the Eye Exhibit, a component of its "Amazing Body Tour," in his honor. Dr. Judianne Kellaway played the key role in the design, construction, content, and presentation of the exhibit, which opened with a black-tie dinner at the museum to honor Ruiz.[19]

In 1997, The University of Texas Board of Regents took notice of Ruiz's tireless efforts and his many professional accomplishments when it named him as the first Distinguished University Chair in the history of The University of Texas System. On September 11, 1997, University of Texas Chancellor Dr. William Cunningham, UT–Houston Health Science Center President, Dr. M. David Low, and other dignitaries gathered at a reception to honor Ruiz as the John S. Dunn Distinguished University Chair in Ophthalmology. The John S. Dunn Foundation contributed $750,000 in a matching formula with the Hermann Eye Fund's $250,000 contribution, creating the endowment and funding the chair "in perpetuity." The Hermann Eye Fund frequently employed this strategy of providing seed money to attract matching funds, which then resulted in the creation of larger grants. The endowment, which grew to over $2 million, was as significant for the

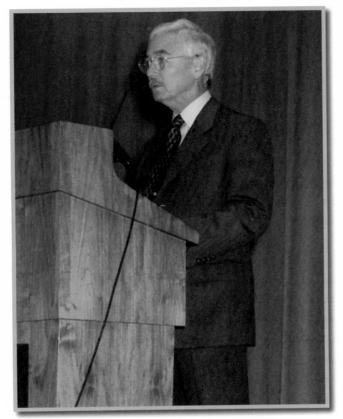

Richard S. Ruiz, MD, at banquet celebrating his appointment to the
first Distinguished University Chair in The University of Texas system,
September 1997.

Department of Ophthalmology and Visual Science, the Medical
School, and the UT–Houston Health Science Center as it was for
Dr. Dick Ruiz. Chancellor Cunningham stressed that endowed
positions gave The University of Texas System the opportunity to
recognize its most outstanding faculty. He stated that "Dr. Ruiz
embodies all the qualities one would hope to find in our faculty" and noted Ruiz's attributes as "a caring physician, dedicated
teacher-mentor, and distinguished scientist." M. David Low acknowledged that he had benefited from Ruiz's skill as one of his
patients and expressed his appreciation for him as "an extraordinary institutional citizen." Low noted the importance of the Vi-

sion Research Consortium and the Basic Science Group to the Medical School, stating that Ruiz had "fostered the development and employment" of those scientists and had "given a home to what I believe will soon be recognized as one of the nation's finest groups of researchers in vision."[20]

Despite these personal and professional triumphs, however, new challenges lay ahead. The health care world in which the Hermann Eye Center existed was going through a series of dramatic changes. The creation of Medicare in 1965 had set in motion a transformation in the way physicians and hospitals provided health care. By the 1980s, the concept of managed care, with its emphasis on integrated systems that offered a full range of health care coverage, had taken hold. The continuing research in medicine and the development of new technology brought new discoveries, new drug treatments, and new diagnostic and surgical techniques. With these advances, however, came increased costs. Changes in government regulations and a huge medical insurance industry affected the delivery of health care, placing increasing financial strains on hospitals in general and on teaching hospitals in particular, which relied heavily upon clinic patients. Increasingly, hospitals searched for new ways to improve cash flow in order to survive. Many hospitals merged with former competitors or created healthcare systems that included locations in affluent areas in order to improve the bottom line. For example, Walter A. Zelman, a former health policy advisor to the Clinton Administration, reported that during 1994, an estimated 176 mergers took place involving some three hundred hospitals, compared to only thirty-two mergers during the previous two years.[21]

In Houston, the situation was no different. In 1962, Memorial Hospital (Memorial Baptist Hospital at that time) had begun developing satellite hospitals in the Houston area while continuing to use its downtown Central Hospital as its network hub. By the mid-1970s, finding that it was land-locked at its downtown location and unable to expand, Memorial built a new flagship hospital in southwest Houston. With the opening of the new facility on January 30, 1977, Memorial closed the downtown hospital and continued expanding its hospital system throughout the area. Over the years, the Memorial Healthcare System had grown to nine hospitals across the greater Houston area, but the system did not have a presence in the Texas Medical Center. Hermann Hospital, with its affiliation as the primary teaching hospital for The University of Texas Medical School at Houston, was in a prestigious Medical Center location and staffed with specialists who could provide state-of-the-art care for even the most seriously ill patients, but it lacked in-depth management expertise and the ability to reach out into the suburbs to expand its private patient base.[22]

During the mid-1990s, St. Luke's Episcopal Hospital and Methodist Hospital explored a possible merger, an effort that failed to come to fruition. Around the same time, merger talks began between Memorial Healthcare System and Hermann Hospital, and on July 1, 1997, the two venerable Houston institutions announced that they would join forces in a merger of the two healthcare systems. The merger meant that the new Memorial Hermann Healthcare System would be the largest non-profit hospital system in the Houston area. The two hospitals, led by Memorial's Chief Executive Officer Dan Wilford and Hermann's Chief Executive Officer David Page, completed the merger on November 4, 1997. Dan Wilford was named as the chief executive of the giant new system, and the final agreement called for both hospitals to have equal representation on the new board. Both hospital systems stood to benefit from the merger, which brought together Memorial's experienced healthcare system managers and a growing network of community hospitals that could refer patients to Hermann for specialized care including its trauma center, burn treatment facilities, transplant center, and the Hermann Eye Center. The Memorial System gained a high-profile hospital in the Texas Medical Center and also a strong affiliation with The University of Texas Medical School. The new Memorial Hermann Healthcare System included nine hospitals,

2,500 patient beds, approximately 11,000 employees, 4,500 physicians, and combined revenues of approximately $2 billion.[23]

Dick Ruiz viewed the merger of the two hospital systems as a positive event. "The merger with the Memorial System has been one of the best things that has happened to Hermann," Ruiz said later. "The Memorial Hermann Hospital System is very strong, probably the strongest in the state, and doing very well." But although the merger created a new system for providing health care in Houston, it also meant that there would be a new administrative model with a new board and new management personnel. Ruiz had known most of the Hermann Hospital Estate's board members and played a role in the hospital's administration as chief of ophthalmology, founding director of the Hermann Eye Center, and chief of staff. But now, new people would be coming along who did not know the Hermann Eye Center, did not know Dick Ruiz, and who were not familiar with the important role he played at the hospital. What all of this meant was not immediately

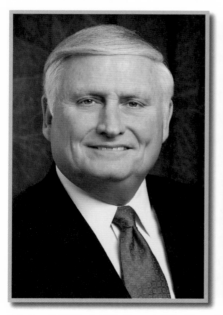 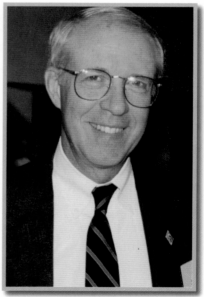

Left, Dan S. Wilford, CEO, Memorial Healthcare System, Courtesy Memorial Hermann Healthcare System. Right, David Page, CEO, Hermann Hospital.

apparent, and for the next few years, the Hermann Eye Center continued to develop as an institution known for its high-quality patient care, teaching, and research.[24]

During this time of merger and changes in administration, Ruiz began thinking about a plan of succession for leadership in the Department of Ophthalmology and Visual Science. In 1999, he chose Dr. Robert M. Feldman as deputy chair of the department. Feldman, an expert in glaucoma, impressed Ruiz with his energy, intelligence, business acumen, skillful patient care, and dedication to the overall mission of the Eye Center. In fact, Ruiz later said that it was Feldman's love of academics and dedication to medicine that led him to recruit Feldman to the program in 1994. Feldman held impressive credentials: a medical degree from Chicago Medical School; a glaucoma research fellowship under Dr. George Spaeth at Wills Eye Hospital in Philadelphia; an internship at New York Infirmary–Beekman Downtown Hospital; a residency at the University of California, San Diego; and a clinical glaucoma fellowship under Dr. Donald Gross at Baylor College of Medicine. In his brief time at The University of Texas Medical School, Feldman was recognized as Outstanding Teacher in Ophthalmology and received the Dean's Excellence Award. In addition to his sterling reputation as a teacher, he had written or co-authored some one hundred book chapters, abstracts, and journal articles on glaucoma re-

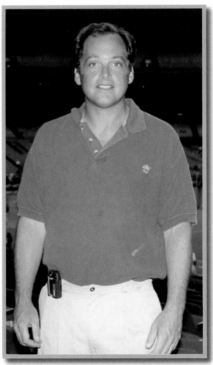

Robert M. Feldman, MD, joined Hermann Eye Center in 1994.

search. At the Hermann Eye Center, Feldman continued his glaucoma research and collaborated with various industry and pharmaceutical companies to test and develop new drug treatments. Feldman also made a point to engage medical students and residents in these projects. "We were able to collaborate and work with industry as well as conduct our own independent projects," said Feldman.

The mission of the Hermann Eye Center—providing the best patient care, teaching students and residents, and the opportunity to conduct research—was a perfect fit for Bob Feldman. "That was all simultaneous as part of the job, being an assistant professor at the time at the Medical School and starting to work in the Eye Center," he recalled later. "And that was really the way the Eye Center was set up: to be working there, you should be a faculty member at the university. The two go hand-in-hand because the two missions go hand-in-hand. It is about practicing medicine but using that practice of medicine for teaching and for clinical research as well." As deputy chair of the department, Feldman had an opportunity to gain valuable experience that would make him a serious candidate to succeed Ruiz when the time came for him to retire as chair.[25]

In November 1999, Dick Ruiz announced that the Eye Center soon would acquire one of the most advanced, FDA-approved systems for laser vision correction. The Hermann Eye Center had been involved with refractive surgery as it evolved over the years, from the introduction of intraocular lenses to the development of radial keratotomy (RK), and later, the introduction of laser vision correction, photorefractive keratectomy (PRK), and the more recent laser-assisted in-situ keratomileusis (LASIK). Through the efforts of Dr. Richard W. Yee, Director of the Cornea Service, and Dr. Nan Wang, MD, PhD, the Hermann Eye Center attempted to develop the new LADARVision® Center, which offered a state-of-the-art instrument to customize the patient's laser vision treatment to the specific needs for each eye with a high level of precision.

Dr. Richard W. Yee, who held the Joe M. Green Chair in Ophthalmology, earned his medical degree at The University of Texas Health Science Center at San Antonio. He had been director of cornea at UT–San Antonio and was internationally known. Since 1994 Yee had been conducting research in corneal dystrophies and molecular biology, looking for the specific genes that caused certain diseases of the eye. His lab was the first NEI-sponsored corneal dystrophy lab approved under the U.S. Department of Health and Human Services Clinical Laboratory Improvement Amendments (CLIA) program. The CLIA program ensures quality laboratory testing through a certification program that is required for the lab to be eligible to receive Medicare or Medicaid payments.

Dr. Nan Wang graduated from Baylor College of Medicine and also earned a PhD in biochemistry from Baylor College of Medicine's Graduate School of Biomedical Science. In addition to her special interests in biochemical and biophysical properties of the eye and her fellowship training in cornea, anterior segment disease, and refractive surgery, Dr. Wang also performed LASIK, PRK, and LASEK surgery to treat myopia, hyperopia, and astigmatism. Although the LA-DARVision® Center later proved to be financially unsustainable, it nevertheless was an example of how the Eye Center continued to seek the most advanced technology to provide the highest level of eye care for patients.[26]

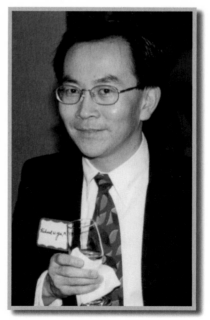

Richard W. Yee, MD, Clinical Professor and Joe M. Green Chair.

While Drs. Feldman and Yee led the Eye Center's clinical research effort, the Basic Science Group was becoming internationally recognized for the excellence of its research. Ruiz continued to seek out highly trained physicians who would bring their specialized skills to the Eye Center. In March 2000, Ruiz convinced Dr. Larry Brenner to come out of his brief retirement to work at the Hermann Eye Center. Brenner had been involved in a four-person ophthalmology practice in Pasadena, where he did most of the ophthalmic plastics and neuro-ophthalmology. Ruiz brought Brenner on board to utilize his skills in the difficult sub-specialty of neuro-ophthalmology. "I strictly do diagnostic work," said Brenner. "It involves serious, vision-loss issues, many of which are not remedial, involving central nervous system problems and systemic problems. They are all thought-provoking, difficult, sometimes perplexing problems." Brenner proved to be an invaluable addition to the Eye Center, providing these specialized services to patients and also teaching medical students, residents, and other physicians who sought training in this complicated subspecialty.[27]

The doctors in the Eye Center continued to explore the latest in ophthalmic diagnostics and treatments. In addition, many of them continued to be involved in clinical research. Ruiz encouraged these endeavors and the Hermann Eye Fund often provided financial assistance to support both the clinical research in the Eye Center and basic science research in the Medical School. Over the years, Ruiz continued to set an example, despite a busy schedule that included seeing patients, teaching, fundraising activities for the Hermann Eye Fund, and his many administrative functions. By the year 2000, Dr. Ruiz had authored or coauthored over seventy-five medical journal articles and delivered over 270 papers, lectures, and presentations across the nation and in such faraway places as Mexico, Canada, Brazil, Argentina, Colombia, Puerto Rico, Peru, and Venezuela.

All of the activities of the Hermann Eye Center temporarily came to a screeching halt the following year, in June 2001, when one of the most devastating weather disasters in Houston's history slammed the area. On June 5, 2001, Tropical Storm Allison

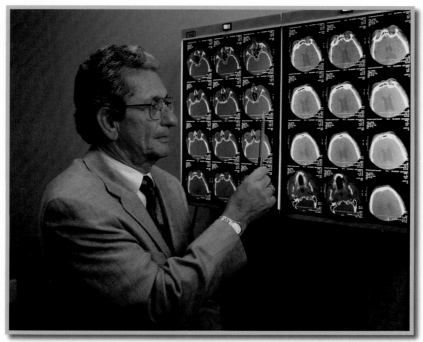

Larry Brenner, MD, teaching neuro-ophthalmology.

formed in the northwest Gulf of Mexico about eighty miles south of Galveston and that evening poured some eight to twelve inches of rain on the greater Houston area. The storm passed through the area, but three days later, the wind currents pushing the storm changed directions and brought Allison back. During the overnight period from Friday, June 8, through the morning of Saturday, June 9, Tropical Storm Allison dumped approximately four inches of rain per hour for about a ten-hour period on the city's already-saturated ground. The massive flooding that followed killed twenty-two people, damaged or destroyed over seventy thousand homes, and caused some $5 billion in damages throughout the Houston area, including about $2 billion in the Texas Medical Center. As a result of the flooding, Hermann Hospital lost electrical power, including its emergency generators. This forced the staff to evacuate all of the hospital's 540 patients. In a heroic effort beginning on Saturday, June 9, and continuing

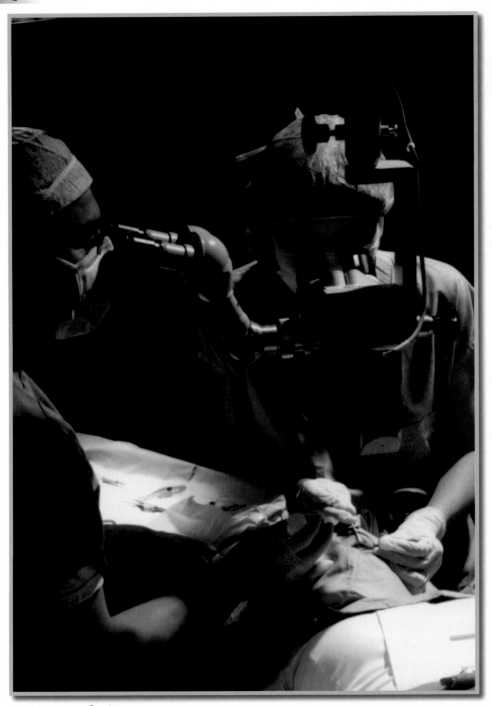

Dr. Nan Wang performing eye surgery.

through the night into Sunday, June 10, approximately three hundred volunteers, including Dick Ruiz and several people from the Eye Center, helped move weary, frightened, and in some cases, desperately ill patients through the hospital's dark corridors and stairwells with only flashlights to show the way.

"All of the emergency generators went out because they were in the basement," Ruiz remembered. "It was a major crisis. The whole medical staff was asked to come help evacuate the patients. I came over along with many others. We had to take these patients down the stairwells and it was pitch black. I will never forget that. They had Hermann Hospital's Life Flight helicopters and also U.S. Army Blackhawk helicopters that came in and helped move these patients out as we would get them down to the street-level emergency center." As the flood waters began to recede, a combination of ambulances and helicopters evacuated patients to hospitals as far as 150 miles away. Although Allison never reached hurricane strength, it is considered the costliest tropical storm ever to hit the United States. [28]

Since both the Hermann Eye Center and the Department of Ophthalmology and Visual Science were on the seventh floor of their respective buildings, they did not suffer from flood damage. But it took several weeks for the initial cleanup and restoration of rudimentary electrical and air conditioning services to both buildings. Hermann Hospital and the Eye Center remained closed for five long weeks, until mid-July. During this time, the Eye Center's administrative staff worked out of the warehouse facilities of the Seasoft Company, a practice management software firm located near the Medical Center, using their cell phones to keep in touch with doctors and patients. Ruiz's former colleagues at Houston Eye Associates and Drs. James Smelley and Charles Garcia graciously made their offices available for the Hermann Eye Center's ophthalmologists to see patients. But in order to see patients, the doctors needed their medical records—the patients' charts—which remained in the Hermann Eye Center's offices on the seventh floor of the Jones Pavilion. The building was without

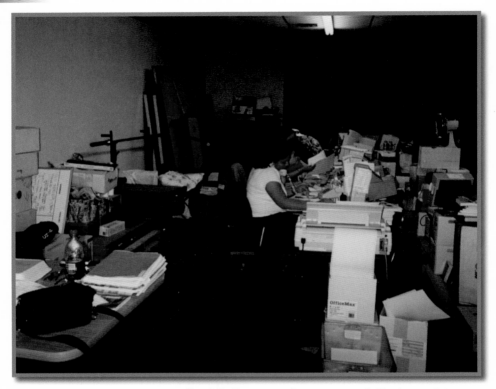

Hermann Eye Center's administrative staff worked off-site, in warehouse space provided by the Seasoft Company, following the devastation of Tropical Storm Allison.

electricity, which also meant no air conditioning, no lighting, and no elevator service. It fell to Sue McRaney, Ramona Singleton, and Eraclio Guzman to make sure that the doctors had their patients' medical records. Every day, they climbed the seven flights of dank, dark stairs, using flashlights to illuminate the way; retrieved patients' charts from the Eye Center's offices; and then trudged through the stifling heat and humidity, back down the steps, carrying the boxes of folders. During this time, McRaney attended daily meetings at Hermann Hospital to receive updates on the recovery effort. The hospital briefly delayed reopening after the electricity was restored because of concerns over the quality of air and water. The Hermann Eye Center reopened in mid-

July, but it would be many months before most of the damaged buildings completely returned to normal.[29]

Having survived the harrowing experience of Tropical Storm Allison, the physicians, staff, faculty, and scientists of the Hermann Eye Center were relieved to return to work and resume their normal routines. As life in the Medical Center began to return to normal in 2002, twenty-five years after he founded the Hermann Eye Center, Dick Ruiz could look back, knowing that his dream of creating a world-class eye center had not only survived a disrupting break-up of the original physician partnership, but also had reemerged stronger than ever, with a team dedicated to fulfilling that purpose. The mission of providing the finest in patient care, teaching, and vision research while operating on a level with the best eye centers in the country is demanding and requires a level of commitment that simply is not for everyone. But Ruiz proved that it could work and found the people who shared his ideas and his level of dedication. In many ways, the first years of the new century seemed to confirm that the Hermann Eye Center had become a permanent institution, something that would last into the foreseeable future as a center of excellence in ophthalmology. But, as always, new challenges were forming behind the scenes and soon the Hermann Eye Center would have to reinvent itself once again in order to perpetuate Ruiz's dream for a comprehensive eye center.

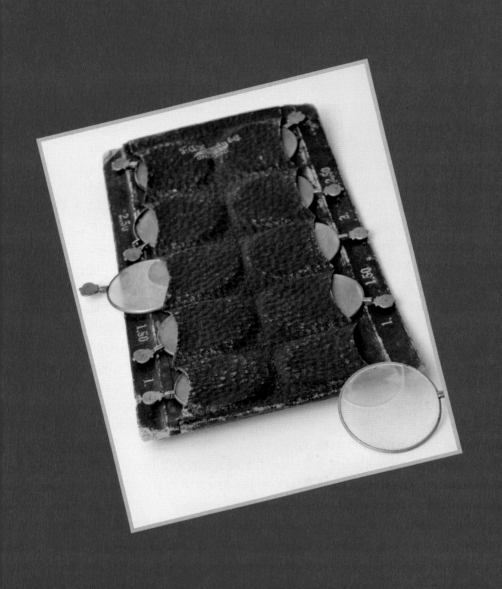

CHAPTER SIX

A New Era, a New Building, and a New Name

I N THE AFTERMATH of Tropical Storm Allison, the Hermann Eye Center's clinical and academic departments enjoyed returning to their normal routines following extensive repairs to their respective buildings. Unknown to anyone, however, events that had begun percolating behind the scenes nearly a decade earlier now threatened to erupt with consequences no one, including Dick Ruiz, could have foreseen. In the end, the clinical arm of the Hermann Eye Center would have a new home, a new name, and the long partnership with Hermann Hospital would change irrevocably.

This amazing turn of events began during the early 1990s, when it first became apparent that Hermann Hospital's Robertson Pavilion needed another extensive renovation. The building, originally constructed in 1949, no longer met Houston's upgraded fire codes. Because of the expense involved to bring the surgical suites and patient rooms into compliance, the Robertson Pavilion was deemed better suited for conversion to office space. Discussions began about a new hospital pavilion, and along with this idea came recognition of the need for a new professional office/outpatient building, with its own day surgery unit, more room for private doctors' offices, and more parking. Dick Ruiz later recalled that during one of the early conversations about the new facility, he made a comment that he would "move the Eye Center into that new outpatient building rather than leave it in the hospital where it really doesn't belong." Ruiz reasoned that as an outpatient service, the clinical arm of the Eye Center was better suited to be in a Hermann Hospital–owned outpatient building than remain within the hospital proper, which was dedicated to inpatient services. He made this observation assuming that the prospective new building would be owned by Hermann Hospital and that the long-standing partnership arrangement with the Eye Center would continue with only minor modifications and in a different space.

Hospital officials and other interested parties met periodically over the next few years to discuss ideas and options. In 1997, however, Hermann Hospital merged with the Memorial Healthcare System, bringing new administrative leadership and a change in the overall management philosophy. Hermann hospital was no longer a stand-alone entity and now had to conform to the priorities and administrative policies of a larger corporate healthcare system. By contrast, the Memorial Healthcare System had little experience operating a teaching hospital or interacting with the academic world of a major medical school. Although it took several years before the ramifications of the merger had a major impact on hospital management, the merger in 1997 signaled the beginning of a new era. In time, the Hermann Eye Center would be caught up in the whirlwind of change created, in part, by the unification with Memorial.

One issue immediately arose in the aftermath of the merger. Memorial Hermann officials knew that the Robertson Pavilion no longer met fire code standards and they now would be required to begin serious planning for the construction of a new hospital building to replace the aging structure. Since a new outpatient building also was badly needed, administrators first explored plans to build them at the same time. This meant that bond financing for the two massive construction projects had to be arranged simultaneously. But the cost for constructing the two buildings was too high to be financed with one bond issue. As there was no choice in the matter, planning for the desperately needed new hospital building, the Hermann Pavilion, moved forward, but plans for the new outpatient building were put on hold. During the next several years, Ruiz had many conversations about the dire need for a new outpatient facility that would include more parking, offices for private doctors who would use Hermann Hospital, an imaging center, an independent day surgery unit, and ample space for facilities to meet other pressing needs. After discussing the issue over a period of time, it was Memorial Hermann Healthcare System's CEO, Dan Wilford, who suggested that instead of relying upon bonds to finance the construction, they should turn to developers in private enterprise who, he astutely noted, "would stand in line to create this new building."[1]

In May 2001, after receiving bids from several firms, Memorial Hermann selected Mischer Healthcare Services as its development partner. Walter Mischer Jr. established Mischer Healthcare Services, a developer of healthcare facilities, in 1994. Prior to that, he had served as chairman of the board of Hermann Hospital Estate and as interim chief executive officer of Hermann Hospital from 1991 to 1993. The board might have chosen him as permanent CEO, but Mischer did not have a formal background in health care administration. According to Ruiz, the board may have seen this as problematic, but he saw it as a huge plus, noting, "Walt Mischer was a proven executive, a success in business, and he loved Hermann Hospital." Indeed, during his term as CEO, Mischer brought a new sense of administrative professionalism, business acumen, and discipline to the hospital and within two years, helped restore Hermann's financial viability in a remarkable turnaround. He and his father, Walter Mischer Sr., who previously had served on the Hermann Hospital Estate's board of trustees, had a long record as successful developers in the greater Houston area. But in June 2001, shortly after Memorial Hermann selected Mischer Healthcare Services as its development partner, Tropical Storm Allison devastated much of Houston, the Texas

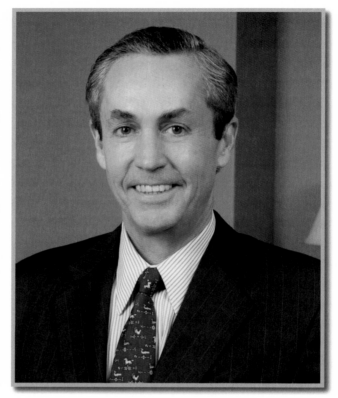

Walter Mischer, Jr. *Courtesy Mischer Healthcare Services*

Medical Center, and Memorial Hermann Hospital, causing a two-year delay in most of the work related to launching the office tower project. Hermann Hospital had suffered more severely than most other hospitals in the Medical Center, sustaining some $100 million in damages. While the hospital was recovering from this disaster, Mischer continued to work in the background on developing plans and seeking investors and tenants in order to line up the financing for the new building. He approached The University of Texas Health Science Center at Houston with a proposal to take an ownership interest in concert with Memorial Hermann as a lead tenant and a limited partner in the new building. With these two medical institutions backing the project, Mischer would have little trouble lining up financing and leasing the remaining space.[2]

On September 10, 2002, officials from Memorial Hermann Healthcare System and The University of Texas Health Science Center at Houston signed a letter of intent to develop a new professional office building and ambulatory care center. It would be the first major building of its kind to be constructed in the Texas Medical Center in about ten years. The plans first called for a twenty-five-story structure to be located on land owned by Memorial Hermann at the northwest corner of the Texas Medical Center, directly across Fannin Street from Memorial Hermann Hospital on the east, and across Main Street from Rice University on the west. Developers planned a signature building of prominent stature for the site, which because of its location on the northern edge facing downtown, was often referred to as the "gateway to the Texas Medical Center." Mischer Healthcare Services would develop the building and also become a general partner in the ownership group. Memorial Hermann and The University of Texas were to be limited partners with lead tenants that included the Hermann Eye Center, The Institute of Rehabilitation and Research, University Care Plus, the UT–Houston Ambulatory Care Center, Memorial Hermann Hospital, and a number of private doctors.[3]

But just as plans for the new building were coming together, in a move that would have serious ramifications for the future of the Hermann Eye Center and also its role in the new professional building, the Memorial Hermann Healthcare System announced a change in leadership. Months earlier, in January 2002, Memorial Hermann's CEO, Dan S. Wilford, announced his retirement. Wilford first joined what then was the Memorial Healthcare System as chief executive officer in 1984. During his eighteen-year tenure, he led the system through an era of unprecedented growth, from three community hospitals to a comprehensive health care network that included ten hospitals and nearly 14,000 employees. Wilford played a key role in the merger of Memorial and Hermann hospitals and helped create the largest not-for-profit health care system in Texas and one of the largest in the country. Now, on October 4, 2002, just a few weeks after the announcement of the UT and Memorial Hermann agreement to develop a new professional office building and ambulatory care center, the board of directors of the Memorial Hermann Healthcare System appointed Daniel J. Wolterman as its president and chief executive officer, succeeding Wilford, who would retire on November 1, 2002. Wolterman, who joined Memorial Hermann in 1999 as senior vice president of hospital operations, had twenty-two years of experience in various executive positions in the healthcare industry, including senior vice president of the Sisters of Charity of the Incarnate Word Health Care System.[4]

Two months after taking over as Memorial Hermann's new president, on January 6, 2003, Wolterman appointed Juanita F. Romans as senior vice president of Memorial Hermann Healthcare System and CEO of Memorial Hermann Hospital (now known as Memorial Hermann Hospital–Texas Medical Center). Romans, who joined Memorial Hermann in 2001, was a highly

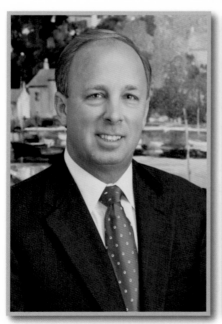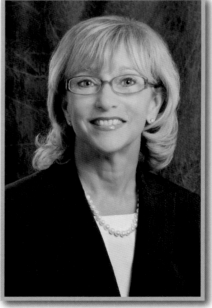

Daniel J. Wolterman, President and CEO, Memorial Hermann Healthcare System. Juanita F. Romans, CEO, Memorial Hermann—Texas Medical Center 2003–10. Courtesy Memorial Hermann Healthcare System

regarded health care professional with some twenty years of clinical and administrative experience. After receiving a nursing degree from the Grace Hospital School of Nursing in Detroit in 1971, Romans began working as a registered nurse. She continued her professional studies, earning a bachelor's degree at the University of Detroit in 1978 and a master's degree in nursing at Wayne State University in 1987. Romans also completed a postgraduate program in health systems management at the Harvard School of Public Health in 1991. Before joining Memorial Hermann, she served as executive vice president at Evanston Northwestern Healthcare in Illinois. [5]

With these new leaders in place, Memorial Hermann Healthcare System and Memorial Hermann Hospital–TMC had a proficient new team of administrators to lead the system and the hospital into a new era of corporate healthcare. However, although Wolterman had been with Memorial Hermann since 1999 and Romans since 2001, neither had near the longevity of Dick Ruiz, nor did they possess the institutional history that would enable them fully to embrace the significance of the hospital's relationship with the Eye Center or to appreciate Ruiz's long-term loyalty to Hermann Hospital.

Just as Wolterman was taking the reins as Memorial Hermann's new president, the deal with The University of Texas Health Science Center to develop a new out-patient office building fell through. Walter Mischer, who was depending upon the UT Health Science Center to be a partner with a sizeable equity position in the new building project, had been developing plans based on the assumption that the Medical School's doctors needed more clinic and office space to see patients under the university's practice plan. As the months passed and Mischer presented multiple design ideas and ownership plans for the new building, it began to appear to some observers that UTHSC–H president James T. Willerson, MD, really wanted the university to have its own medical office building. In the end, after considering a series of options including a separate tower, designated elevators to UT-owned floors, and even a condominium-style ownership plan, The University of Texas determined that it could not or would not participate in any of these ownership proposals.[6]

No doubt disappointed by the withdrawal of The University of Texas from the agreement, Mischer continued to recruit private investors. By the spring of 2003, he also had assembled a list of potential tenants and developed an innovative new plan for financing. He remembered that Ruiz had said he would move the Hermann Eye Center to an outpatient facility, and asked early on if he still remained interested in the idea. As Ruiz recalled later, "I was naively thinking that it was going to be owned by the hospital and therefore the relationship with the Eye Center would remain unchanged. Well, of course, it didn't develop that way." Ruiz answered in the affirmative, making a commitment that became an important element to the deal. Mischer needed to have a little more than 30 percent of the building pre-leased in order to get financing for the construction. "We were a real key player to the success of that thing," said Ruiz, "to commit early that we would go in there and take at least one whole floor. I pretty much stuck my neck way out there. And the hospital ... I think, ended up with four floors. So then there were five floors guaranteed." As Mischer later observed, Ruiz's commitment "was a real turning point for the building's success." When Dr. Paul Cook agreed to take about half of the nineteenth floor for his OB/GYN practice and Ruiz committed to another section of the same floor, enough of the building was pre-leased to meet the requirements for financing the project. "That pushed us over the threshold," said Mischer.[7]

Originally, Walter Mischer had presented an enticing offer to Ruiz, stating that the Eye Center could have the same deal he had offered to UT and own an entire floor of the building. But, with UT pulling out of the deal, it did not make sense to have one tenant owning only one floor. Ruiz and Mischer then agreed on a different ownership plan. "So, then we ended up just leasing like everybody else," said Ruiz. "But we also invested $5 million of Eye Fund money for a significant equity position in that building." Mischer's unique plan brought together Memorial Hermann Healthcare System (with about a 45 percent stake in the building), outside investors—prominent Houston businessmen—and later, doctors who planned to lease space in the building and who were offered the option to buy limited equity on a formula basis. Although not many doctors were able to accept this unique offer, the idea of potentially holding some equity in the building proved to be a great marketing tool and brought many in as tenants. Those doctors who did opt to take an equity share had the same opportunity as the major investors to realize a return on the building and possibly could look forward to a handsome profit upon its future sale. Dick Ruiz calculated that, in addition to being a stellar investment opportunity for the Eye Fund, the cash flow generated once the building was fully occupied would help to offset a significant portion of the rental costs for the Eye Clinic.[8]

As plans for the new building moved forward, Ruiz sought confirmation that Memorial Hermann would continue its long-standing partnership with the Hermann Eye Center. Since the Eye Center would be vacating 35,000 square feet of space within the hospital to move its clinic across the street, Ruiz and hospital officials needed to reach an agreement on the future of the partnership. The primary question related to what future role Hermann Hospital would play as a partner with the Eye Center. In conjunction with this was the Eye Center's commitment to provide care for the hospital's indigent eye patients, its use of hospital facilities for inpatient treatment and surgery, and the around-the-clock emergency room coverage and consultation. Throughout its history, the Eye Center's physicians had provided these services and Hermann Hospital had provided clinic space in the Jones Pavilion for the Eye Center's clinic. Another remaining question was to what extent the hospital would provide assistance with the move. Finally, would the hospital continue to provide administrative services, at the same cost, for the staff employees at the Eye Center?

Ruiz began a series of extensive correspondence and meet-

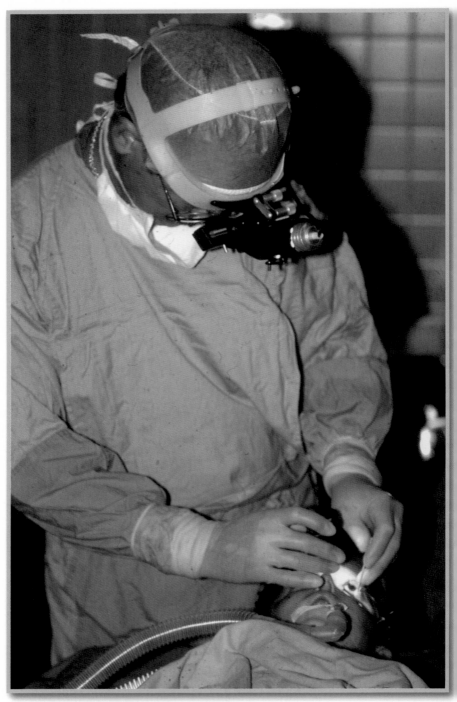

Dr. Ruiz examining a child under general anesthesia.

ings with Juanita Romans and Dan Wolterman, first to provide background history on the Hermann Eye Center and then to discuss specific terms of the continuing partnership. Ruiz had no doubt that the relationship would continue, but the nature and extent of that affiliation surely would change. He wrote to Wolterman in advance of their first meeting, scheduled for May 28, 2003, to provide a brief history of the Eye Center and its partnership with the hospital. Ruiz emphasized the "unique and loyal partnership that has lasted twenty-six years, between the Hospital, the ophthalmologists of the Hermann Eye Center, The University of Texas, and the Hermann Eye Fund." He noted that the only cost to the hospital during that time was to provide space for the Eye Center. By contrast, the Eye Center had "contributed in many ways" to both Hermann and, later, Memorial Hermann, by attracting patients, by enhancing the reputation of the hospital for providing the finest in medical care, and by helping the hospital fulfill its responsibilities to provide care for indigent patients. In addition, the Hermann Eye Fund had provided "hundreds of thousands of dollars' worth of eye equipment and instruments for the Hospital." Ruiz also stated the current dilemma that the Eye Center would now face: the high rent for space in the new building, a fee that would be beyond its means to afford. "We would like for Memorial Hermann to continue to be our partner," concluded Ruiz. "I ask you to consider how Memorial Hermann can help financially with this move." Following their initial meeting, Wolterman wrote to Ruiz stating, "I look forward to continuing the mutually beneficial relationship of our two organizations. It goes without saying that I appreciate your support and commitment to Memorial Hermann. If I can ever be of any assistance to you, please do not hesitate to call me."[9]

Although its language was not specific, Wolterman's note seemed to affirm that the Eye Center and Memorial Hermann would continue their partnership. Ruiz sought clarification and again summarized the relationship between the Eye Center and the Hospital in a memorandum to Juanita Romans a few days later.

"The pertinent question," Ruiz wrote, was, "What role will Memorial Hermann Hospital play in the future of the [Hermann] Eye Center?" He reiterated that in 1975, the Hermann Hospital Estate Board of Trustees had voted unanimously to dedicate space to an Eye Center. The resulting partnership with Hermann Hospital, University Eye Associates, donors to the Hermann Eye Fund, and The University of Texas Department of Ophthalmology and Visual Science proved to have been very successful. "We need to define the future role of Memorial Hermann as a partner," stated Ruiz. "It would be my preference for the Eye Center to continue to be owned by Memorial Hermann and the name changed to Memorial Hermann Eye Center." Ruiz pointed out several important ways that Memorial Hermann Hospital would benefit from this arrangement. The fact that the Eye Center was vacating the entire seventh floor of the Jones Pavilion opened up some 35,000 square feet of space for hospital use. In addition to the newly available space, Memorial Hermann would continue to profit from the international reputation of the Eye Center. The hospital would gain financially from use of its facilities for eye patient care and from the Eye Center's delivery of indigent patient care which the hospital was obligated to provide under George Hermann's will and under a 1985 mandate from the Attorney General of the State of Texas following an investigation into Hermann Hospital's charity practices.

Ruiz also noted that while he was asking Memorial Hermann to invest financially in the Eye Center, "the entire investment, plus appreciation, will be recouped at the point of sale." Additionally all improvements paid for by Hermann Eye Fund would accrue to the hospital.[10]

Despite Dick Ruiz's artful presentation over a period of several months, on September 2, 2003, Juanita Romans informed him that Memorial Hermann Hospital had decided not to continue the partnership with the Hermann Eye Center once it finally moved to the new Memorial Hermann Medical Plaza. "I do not understand the rationale for the decision," Ruiz later wrote in a letter to Dan Wolterman. "For example, if the main reason for refusing my proposal entails the System needing to raise additional investment dollars, we can work that out. Should we discuss the matter further?"[11]

But times had changed. In the aftermath of the Memorial and Hermann merger, the new institution, by virtue of its size and nature, had a new modus operandi. The world of health care continued to evolve into a more complex arena filled with multiple layers of hospital administrators, insurance company bureaucrats, hosts of lawyers, and the federal government. The era had passed in which a venerable private hospital and a highly regarded physician could effect a "gentlemen's agreement" with a memorandum and a handshake. In its place came healthcare systems with new priorities, collective needs, and the requirement to achieve "systemness" by transforming all units into a common identity.

In the wake of this unforeseen and surprising turn of events, Ruiz began quickly to formulate a new plan for the future of the Eye Center. He had faced similar obstacles before, but this time he had plenty of resources which he could employ as he charted the future course for the Eye Center. The Hermann Eye Center had become a highly respected institution, known internationally for leading the way in patient care and for its excellent training program for ophthalmologists. It also had a firm reputation for clinical research, and the Department of Ophthalmology and Visual Science, with its Basic Science Group, continued to build a sterling record in academics and laboratory research. In addition, the Hermann Eye Fund provided a financial mechanism that enabled Ruiz and the Hermann Eye Center to enjoy a measure of autonomy and freedom that extended beyond the usual bureaucratic restrictions of the hospital and the medical school. As chief of ophthalmology at Memorial Hermann Hospital, chair of the Department of Ophthalmology and Visual Science at The University of Texas Medical School at Houston, founding director of the Hermann Eye Center, and president of the Hermann Eye Fund, Ruiz also had a high measure of personal stature that gave him entrée to philanthropic foundations and access to individuals who had long supported his concept of building an exceptional eye center at Memorial Hermann Hospital.

Ruiz prepared to launch a new fundraising campaign to provide the financial resources he would need to build out the new space and create an endowment that would secure the future for the Eye Center. During the mid-1970s he had realized the goal of raising $2 million to build out the seventh floor of the Jones Pavilion. Now, he had a far more ambitious and risky undertaking, with a goal of $8.5 million. But, as he prepared to launch the "Vision for the Future" campaign, some of the long-time supporters of the Hermann Eye Fund wondered out loud why the Eye Center had to move at all. Had not the original arrangement worked well and to everyone's benefit since 1977? In a letter written March 25, 2004, Ruiz asked Juanita Romans for a clear statement by the hospital. Ruiz could not launch his fundraising campaign while many of his benefactors still held this unanswered question.[12]

Romans's response mirrored the new priorities of the fast-growing Memorial Hermann Healthcare System (MHHS). This communiqué is something of a landmark document in that it reiterated the fact that Hermann Hospital was no longer a "stand-alone hospital," a factor that ultimately led to this "significant, perhaps even monumental change for the Hermann Eye Center." Romans stated that Memorial Hermann Hospital was the only hospital in the MHHS where an entire floor was devoted to a legally separate and distinct clinical program. Now that the hospital was part of a larger entity, the time had come for it to conform to the overall goals of the system. In other words, what once had been a mutually beneficial arrangement had outlived its usefulness. "This has been a concern of ours, or so I'm told, from the very initiation of the merger in 1997," said Romans. "However, the long-standing relationship between the Eye Center and the hospital justified our moving slowly rather than rapidly to effect change." The administrators of the Memorial Hermann Healthcare System viewed the construction of the new outpatient professional building as an opportunity to make another stride toward its goal of "systemness," and for the Eye Center to take what they viewed as the "inevitable" step of moving to a new home. "We have nothing but the highest regard for the great contributions of the Hermann Eye Center to both Hermann Hospital and the community it serves," Romans concluded, "and we hope that your benefactors will continue to generously support the Eye Center and the Hermann Eye Fund."[13]

In the midst of all these communications with the hospital, Ruiz received some unexpected good news regarding the academic arm of the Eye Center. The UT System Board of Regents announced that it had voted unanimously to change the name of the ophthalmology department to the Richard S. Ruiz, MD, Department of Ophthalmology and Visual Science upon his retirement as chair of the department. In a statement, the dean of the Medical School, Stanley Schultz, MD, expressed his pleasure that the board of regents had decided to honor Dick Ruiz. "Dr. Ruiz has done so much for the Medical School, and this is a way that the Medical School can show its gratitude."[14]

With this news providing something of a psychological boost, Ruiz and his staff began to work out the specific details of the move. After all of the letters, e-mails, and meetings, Ruiz concluded that most of the Memorial Hermann administrative staff was too young to know about the history and background of the Hermann Eye Center. Since Hermann Hospital had been absorbed into a large, corporate system, the history of its partnership with the Eye Center had been forgotten, making it easier to set that relationship aside. Now, however, there were practical business ramifications that came into play and questions that no longer could be ignored. It is important to note that Hermann Hospital's primary role in the partnership with the Eye Center was to furnish the physical home, while the Eye Center provided ophthalmic care on a twenty-four hour, 365-day-a-year basis for the indigent patients that came to Hermann Hospital's emergency room. Eye Center physicians also provided consultations and attended to an increasing number of cases in the emergency room that were referred from outlying hospitals, including the other member hospitals of the Memorial Hermann System; many of these cases were uninsured, indigent patients. "We were happy to do all this indigent care, which included running the indigent outpatient clinic," said Ruiz, "and cover all these things, because the quid pro quo was that we were provided with a beautiful eye center for patient care." But now that the Eye Center would be moving out of the Memorial Hermann Jones Pavilion and into space for which it had to pay high rent, new questions arose about how to compensate the Eye Center's physicians for these services to the hospital. As Ruiz remembered, "We had never asked them for a penny. As a matter of fact, it was the opposite. I used to support the hospital by buying microscopes, surgical equipment, and all sorts of things with Eye Fund money, the justification being that we were a training program for residents, fellows, nurses, techs, and medical students; we were taking care of indigent patients; and we were doing research."[15]

One option available to the Eye Center was to take legal action and force the issue with the Hospital. Although there was no contract, per se, between the Eye Center and the Hospital, there were memoranda, official minutes from Hermann Hospital Estate Board meetings, and other documents that would have made the case for the Center to insist on staying in the Jones Pavilion, or to insist that Memorial Hermann provide an equivalent facility in one of its other buildings. In the end, however, this was not a course that Ruiz ever considered. He had been steadfastly loyal to Hermann Hospital throughout his entire career. Although the recent turn of events was not what he anticipated, the deep regard—bordering on reverence—that he held for the hospital, along with his own practical nature, precluded any course of action that might develop into hostility.[16]

But that same realistic nature brought Ruiz to ask the Hospital to pay the costs of the move. Ruiz again wrote to Juanita Romans, asking that Memorial Hermann provide financial assistance. By this time, Ruiz and Romans had held many meetings and began to see eye-to-eye on a number of issues that affected both the Eye Center and Memorial Hermann Hospital. Romans agreed that the Hospital would cover the moving expenses and also began discussions about a new agreement to cover the Eye Center's costs for providing professional services for indigent care, emergency services, and consultations. While the Eye Center bore the brunt of eye patient "dumping" from other local hospitals, Memorial Hermann–TMC experienced the same phenomenon in a much broader and costlier sense. Hospitals throughout the System and others across the region regularly sent trauma patients and most of their indigent patients to Memorial Hermann–TMC. The hospital gladly provided medical care for these patients, but there was no way that it could afford to do this indefinitely without receiving fair financial compensation from the sending hospitals. This shared burden helped open the lines of communication and, in time, led to a new arrangement between the Eye Center and Memorial Hermann Hospital.[17]

During the next few months, the pace of events began to quicken. On September 1, 2004, Memorial Hermann Healthcare System and The University of Texas Health Science Center at Houston reached an historic agreement. The Health Science Center would pay $31 million to purchase the Hermann Professional Building, which originally had been built in 1949, and rename it The University of Texas Health Science Center Professional Building. Along with the acquisition of the building, the Health Science Center renewed its commitment to use Memorial Hermann Hospital as its primary private teaching hospital for an additional fifteen years. The agreement gave the Health Science Center its own building and identity for outpatient clinic space and gave the Memorial Hermann System significant capital to continue its expansion efforts. Before agreeing to the sale of the Hermann Professional Building, Memorial Hermann briefly considered the notion of creating different partnership agreements that would have tied the two projects together with the potential for offering two classes of space for potential tenants: the older

Hermann Professional Building or the more prestigious (and more expensive) Medical Plaza. Eventually, the site could be redeveloped with the addition of a hotel, another professional building, a residential condominium component, and more parking. As Walter Mischer observed, "The site is big enough and there was a lot of flexibility in what you could do with it." But in the end, a partnership with The University of Texas proved to be too difficult and Memorial Hermann agreed to sell the older building. "It turned out all right," Mischer later observed, "but it didn't optimize the asset [property]."[18]

Later in September, officials from Mischer Healthcare Services and Memorial Hermann Healthcare System held groundbreaking ceremonies for the new professional building, to be named Memorial Hermann Medical Plaza (MHMP). The project would be the largest new commercial construction project in the city and would involve a capital investment of some $155 million. With 500,000 rentable square feet and a 2,400-vehicle parking garage, the new structure would be the largest medical office building in the Texas Medical Center. Located directly across Fannin Street from Memorial Hermann Hospital–TMC, the new facility would include an ambulatory care center and a lobby-concourse with space for retail shops and restaurants. The new building would be connected by a sky bridge over Fannin Street to the Memorial Hermann Hospital and topped with a distinctive, sixty-foot "lantern." Dan Wolterman, CEO of the Memorial Hermann System, stated that the new building would attract "the best and brightest in Houston's medical community. It represents, once again, our system's leadership commitment to innovation."[19]

The Memorial Hermann Medical Plaza's exceptional location, innovative design, and unique features all would contribute to make the building a true Houston landmark. As Walter Mischer explained, the opportunity to develop one of the last vacant sites in the Texas Medical Center, a site that truly was "institutional-quality real estate," also carried a tremendous responsibility. As he later observed, "From a design standpoint, you don't want, either architecturally or functionally, to under-design a building for a world-class site like that." Mischer noted that the design process consisted of several levels of planning. One aspect involved the infrastructure of the building, its "floor plate design," in which the architects and engineers had to consider the special requirements and needs for an out-patient medical office building, including clinical space, corridors, physicians' offices and exam rooms, special procedure rooms that might require certain types of mechanical, electrical, and cooling specifications, and also the need for administrative areas. A second level of design involved the structural integrity of the building as contrasted to a standard office building. Most tall buildings are designed to sway slightly in the wind, but a medical tower had to be constructed to meet tighter specifications. "Structurally, it has to be beefed up to a point where it cannot vibrate or sway," said Mischer. "You have to stiffen it through the use of steel and concrete." In addition to the internal design of the building, the exterior look—the shape, size, height, number of floors, and how it would fit on the site—was key to the success of the project.

To meet these design challenges, Mischer selected the Kirksey architectural firm. Mischer credits Robert C. "Bob" Inaba, the firm's executive vice president and director of design, for many of the innovative features of the Memorial Hermann Medical Plaza. "Bob made a lot of contributions to it but in particular, the curtain wall as they call it: the exterior glass system with its innovative use of frets—little strips of sandblasted areas on the interior of the glass that reflect the light." With this type of glass, as the sun moves during the day or if the sky becomes cloudy, the glass reflects the light in a way that causes the building to seem to change its exterior color. In addition to this creative use of special glass, the roof of the building includes a lantern-type structure that rises fifty-three feet. It is made up of a trapezoid design in the middle with reflective surfaces and is surrounded by fifty-six LED light fixtures of different colors mounted on the roof that illuminate it at night. The lights offer a color palette that allows the building's managers to change the colors for special events and holidays.[20]

The D. E. Harvey Builders construction company began work on the Medical Plaza in October 2004. The Medical Plaza and the new Hermann Pavilion were just two projects in a massive building campaign that ultimately included major construction or renovations on all nine MHHS campuses. In order to pay for all of these projects, Memorial Hermann utilized the innovative means of financing pioneered with the Medical Plaza building. Marshall Heins, vice president of construction, real estate, and support services for Memorial Hermann, explained, "It's a new era, I believe, for not-for-profit systems to go out and seek for-profit partners to help us develop so we can devote our capital to our core business, which is providing health care to the community." Heins stated that Memorial Hermann contributed the land for the Medical Plaza and held about 45 percent equity in the massive building. Mischer Healthcare Services raised the additional equity through a private placement offering and by offering tenants, including the Hermann Eye Center, the opportunity to invest in the project. "It's an effort to help them have some return on their investment to help offset occupancy costs and hopefully have a good return once the building has appreciated," Heins said. The thirty-story building was scheduled to be completed in 2006.[21]

With construction of the new building underway, Ruiz stepped up the Hermann Eye Fund's "Vision for the Future" campaign to raise $8.5 million. On the Eye Center's website, Ruiz stated, "The new Eye Center will provide easy access with convenient parking and be designed specifically to serve eye patients, support research, and train ophthalmologists. I hope you will share our 'Vision for the Future' and consider a generous gift so that the Eye Center can continue to be a world leader in ophthalmology, vision research, patient care, and education." He planned for $1.5 million to build out and furnish the new space for the Hermann Eye Center; $5 million would be dedicated to underwrite the cost of continuing and expanding the Eye Center's indigent care, teaching, and research; and $2 million would be set aside to endow a

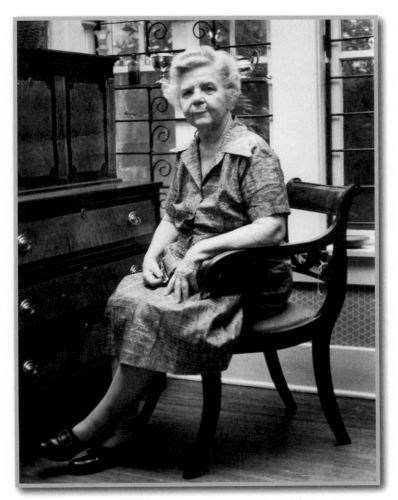

Elizabeth Morford, who earned a national reputation as an expert in American antiques, left her estate to the Hermann Eye Fund.

new position within The University of Texas: Director of Clinical Research in the Department of Ophthalmology and Visual Science at The University of Texas Medical School at Houston.[22]

It is important to note the significance of the Eye Fund as one of the fundamental blocks upon which Ruiz built the Hermann Eye Center. With it he also established an almost unheard-of degree of autonomy within both Memorial Hermann Hospital and The University of Texas Medical School at Houston. Ruiz had created the Eye Fund back in 1968 to help offset the cost of providing eye care for indigent patients and to provide the latest high tech instrumentation not only for patient care but also for teaching. During the mid-1970s, he raised some $2 million when he founded the Hermann Eye Center to fund the build-out of the space in the hospital's Jones Pavilion. Over the years, many foundations, wealthy philanthropists, and grateful eye patients contributed to the Eye Fund. One of the most generous donations came in 1980 from Miss Elizabeth Morford, who gave $125,000 to help equip the minor surgery suite, which was then named the Elizabeth Morford Eye Day Surgery Unit. Morford graduated from Rice Institute in 1921 with honors in chemistry and biology. When her mother died in 1929, she gave up her career in the sciences and took over her mother's small business, the Green Bottle Antique Shop. During the next fifty years, Morford became one of the most successful and highly regarded antique dealers specializing in Americana, for which she was nationally known. When she died in September 1983, unbeknownst to Dick Ruiz or the Eye Center staff, she bequeathed some $1 million to the Hermann Eye Fund. "She never said anything to me," Ruiz remembered. "But about a month or two after she died, I got a call from a lawyer who said that she had left the bulk of her estate to the Hermann Eye Fund. It amounted to over one million dollars, primarily in antiques and property."[23]

Throughout the history of the Eye Fund, Dick Ruiz had been a shrewd and diligent manager. Through his stewardship, the Fund continued to grow and served as a valuable financial resource for all components of the Eye Center. Dr. Tom Prager, who joined the Eye Center in 1979, observed that the Eye Fund "is the strength in the department—teaching, research, patient care—it subsidizes all of that." Because the Eye Fund consistently played a key role in supporting the mission of the Hermann Eye Center, enthusiastic supporters provided a steady flow of donations over the years.[24]

During 2006, as the "Vision for the Future" campaign was developing, Robert Cizik, a retired business executive, dropped a bombshell on Dick Ruiz. Cizik had served as president, chief executive officer, and chairman of the board of Cooper Industries, Inc., from 1973 to 1996. Following his retirement, Cizik and members of his family, who were longtime patients of Ruiz, continued to serve on a number of corporate boards and created a family foundation as a means of supporting various charitable organizations in the community. When Ruiz asked if he would help with the "Vision for the Future" campaign, Cizik replied that he would discuss the matter with his family. Like many fundraising campaigns, the "Vision for the Future" had certain named levels at which donors could contribute and receive recognition, including "naming rights" for certain components of the Eye Center. When Cizik contacted Ruiz again, he stated that he would support the fundraising campaign and offered two options, a token gift or a larger contribution, the level at which he would be recognized with naming rights for the new clinic. "Which would you prefer?" he asked. Apparently, the generous offer was a bit of a shock to Ruiz, who later recalled, "He made this wonderful, generous gesture, and equally important to me was that he is a very upstanding, well-respected gentleman with an impeccable reputation. I said I would be honored to have his name on the clinic." Cizik's pledge was vital to the success of the "Vision for the Future" campaign and enabled Ruiz to focus more attention on the design and build-out of the new eye clinic.[25]

In December 2006, D. E. Harvey Builders completed construction work on the Memorial Hermann Medical Plaza. The build-out and finishing of interior space continued into 2007. The new structure, the tallest medical office building in the Texas Medical Center, had taken about two and a half years and involved some 3,000 people in its construction. With a total of 1.5 million square feet of space, the thirty-story tower represented a capital investment of approximately $157.5 million. "Memorial Hermann Medical Plaza is truly a world-class health care facility," said developer Walter Mischer. The building had the latest in amenities, including "smart building" components, a flexible planning grid, and ownership opportunities for tenants. The new Ambulatory

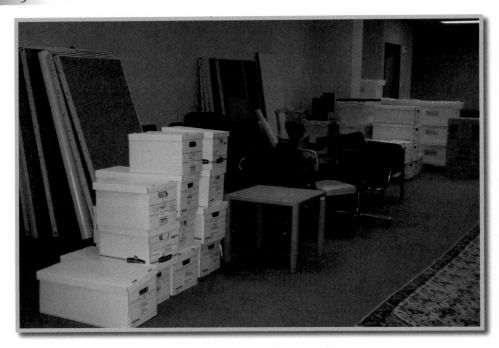

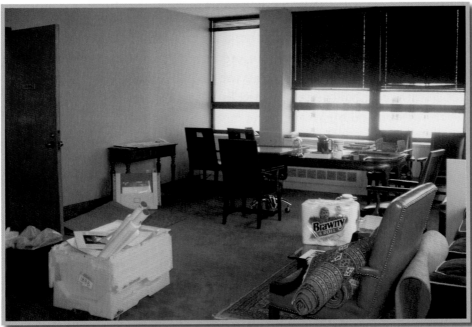

Top, boxes and crates ready for moving. Bottom, Ruiz's office, packed and ready for the movers.

Care Center occupied 100,000 square feet and included the Ambulatory Surgery Center, an Imaging Center, and the Institute for Sports Medicine and Human Performance, which was described as "the largest, most comprehensive, medical-based sports program in the Southwest."[26]

After almost thirty years in the same location, the Hermann Eye Center staff prepared to move the eye clinic (now known as the Robert Cizik Eye Clinic), into the new Memorial Hermann Medical Plaza during the weekend of June 29–July 1, 2007. Although the move was a short distance—just across Fannin Street—it was a major challenge to pack and haul the sensitive instruments and heavy equipment, furniture, art, patient records, and other paraphernalia involved with operating a major eye clinic. Sue McRaney stepped forward and took charge of planning and organizing the logistics of relocating to the new building.

McRaney had a number of issues to resolve in planning the move, foremost of which was the logistics of hauling the physical assets across a very busy Fannin Street, which ran through the heart of the Texas Medical Center. Choosing a time that would be most efficient and the least disruptive was the first challenge. McRaney concluded that the move could be accomplished over a weekend and that the clinic could be operational in time to see patients on the following Monday morning. Coordinating a move of this magnitude was challenging, because there were so many items and individuals involved. In the end, a team that included people from the Eye Center, Memorial Hermann Hospital, Mischer Healthcare Services, and a small army of technicians, vendors, and movers developed a comprehensive moving plan that included arrangements for moving and installation of audio/visual equipment, copiers, servers, computers, and telephones in the new offices. Then there was the liquidation of old furniture and equipment, new parking arrangements, overseeing of the floor plan, and acquisition of new furniture to worry about. Even the vending machines had to be relocated. Several professional firms joined the effort, including relocation consultants Leslie

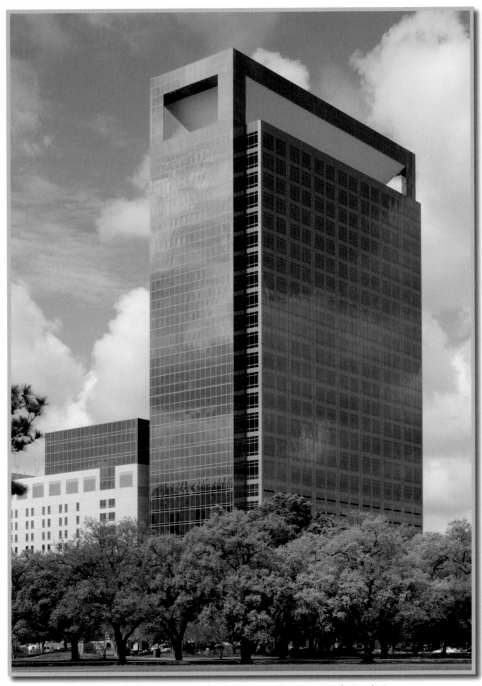

Memorial Hermann Medical Plaza, new home for the Hermann Eye Center/Cizik Eye Clinic.

and Associates. McRaney contracted with Lombart Instruments, the firm that supplied much of the Eye Center's equipment over the years, including exam chairs, stands, and slit lamps, to move that equipment. Pioneer Moving Company moved the other heavy items, including file cabinets, patient records, and office equipment. Sue McRaney recalled later, "As we got down to it, it was pretty well organized. The movers brought in the moving crates. Everybody had a number and a moving kit, so we put our numbers on the crates and packed whatever we wanted in them. At the last, it just got to be ridiculous, because after thirty years, there was so much stuff. But, we somehow managed."[27]

Although most moves involved loading items in large trucks for the journey, since the new building was just across the street and connected by a sky bridge walkway to the hospital, it seemed that the sky bridge would be a sensible option for moving some of the lighter and more sensitive equipment. However, the property managers insisted that hauling boxes and equipment across the sky bridge was not a viable option, because they did not want moving activities to disrupt the retail corridor in the new building. But McRaney, thinking on her feet, asked if they could just move the artwork across the sky bridge and through the corridor. The movers had instructions to be as invisible as possible coming through the retail concourse. The scheme worked so well that they continued using the walkway to move the most fragile instruments and ophthalmic equipment.

The move involved the entire staff of the Hermann Eye Center, some of whom had been with Dick Ruiz for a long time and others who were recent additions. But all joined the effort and did their share in what was a labor-intensive and somewhat emotional endeavor. On Friday evening, the final day that they would be located in the Jones Pavilion, Sue McRaney recalled that, although it was growing late, "Dr. Ruiz was still there. And so, the front [area] people had brought some wine and cheese and grapes and they found a place to set it up. Then they brought him over and toasted him. It was really sweet. He was going to try to make

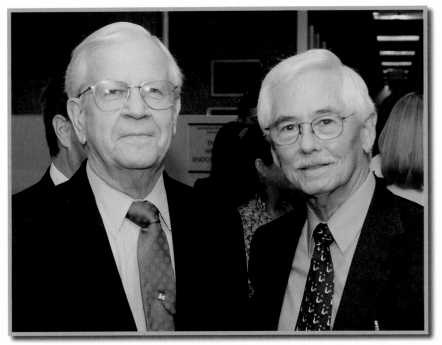

Robert Cizik and Richard Ruiz at the grand opening of the Cizik Eye Clinic in the Memorial Hermann Medical Plaza.

a little talk and he didn't make it through without the tears."[28]

The massive effort by his staff to accomplish the move was not lost on Ruiz, who gratefully observed, "The move went just about as smoothly as possible and it still was a monumental task ... there was just so much stuff, so many file cabinets, so much paper. The records alone—I don't know—300,000 records. Sue McRaney put in about eighty hours a week for probably the last six weeks with this move. It really has been incredible. And all of the employees really chipped in and helped." The move continued through the weekend and by Monday morning, July 2, the Robert Cizik Eye Clinic opened in its new home, on the eighteenth floor of the Memorial Hermann Medical Plaza. "We weren't completely together," said Sue McRaney. "There were still a few things undone. But we had telephones and we had computers up ... and we had the medical records. A lot of us put in some Saturdays and

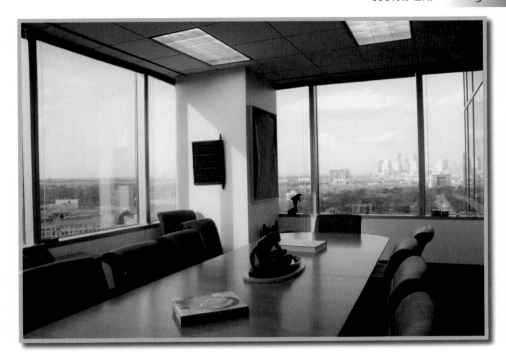

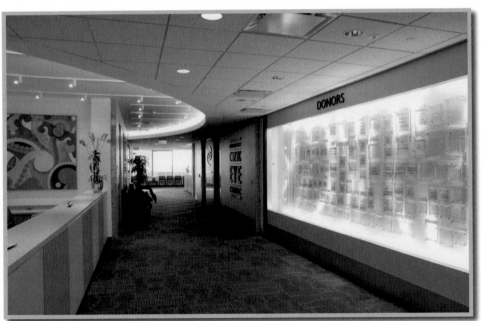

Top, Cizik Eye Clinic conference room and view looking north. Bottom, Donor Wall—Cizik Eye Clinic—designed by Kirk Baxter.

Sundays and a good many hours on that weekend, but it got done and it was a very interesting process."[29]

Approximately three hundred guests, including friends, supporters, and Hermann Eye Fund board members, joined Dick Ruiz on October 30, 2007, for the official grand opening of the Robert Cizik Eye Clinic. The new facilities, which occupied the entire eighteenth floor of the Memorial Hermann Medical Plaza, had the most sophisticated equipment available for patient care. The nineteenth floor was the location for the Raye and Ed White Conference Center, which included a sixty-six seat lecture hall equipped with state-of-the-art audiovisual equipment, a conference room, and kitchen facilities, all dedicated to the Eye Center's mission of teaching and research. Although the new eye clinic was not "contiguous" to the Medical School as was the Jones Pavilion, it was only slightly more distant—just across the street—and remained physically connected via the sky bridge to the hospital and the Medical School. The physicians of University Eye Associates continued to hold clinical faculty appointments in the Department of Ophthalmology and Visual Science, and the mission of the Eye Center—to foster the best in patient care, education, and research—remained the same.

Thirty years after it first opened, Dick Ruiz had once again successfully reinvented the Eye Center. Throughout its history, the core mission and values remained constant, as did Ruiz's idea of a comprehensive, world-class eye center in Houston. Relocating the clinical arm of the center meant the end of the partnership with Memorial Hermann Hospital and tested Ruiz's mettle as an entrepreneur. The decision to invest in the new building as both an owner and tenant was innovative and bold. Although larger in scope than the challenges he had faced previously, Ruiz believed that the potential benefits of investing in the new building far outweighed the prospects for failure. As he had always done, Ruiz gathered the information, analyzed the facts, and made the decision to participate in the project. Financially, the decision to move represented an enormous risk. But, when Robert Cizik, and later, Mary Johnston, Louisa Sarofim, Will Farish, and others presented their generous contributions to the Eye Fund, they also provided the base on which to build the "Vision for the Future" campaign and the momentum to sustain it to a successful conclusion. Thus, the decision to move and the ensuing fundraising campaign also opened the door for Ruiz to put the Eye Center on a more independent financial basis that would ensure its survival long into the future.

Ironically, the move into the Memorial Hermann Medical Plaza physically placed Dick Ruiz almost back to where he began his career forty-five years earlier: next-door to the old Hermann Professional Building. Although the distance from building to building was short, Ruiz had traveled a long way in his quest to build the Eye Center. Gazing out from the Cizik Eye Clinic's beautiful offices to the spectacular view of downtown Houston, Rice University, Hermann Park, and the Texas Medical Center below, Ruiz finally could afford to savor the moment. He had achieved his dream of creating one of the country's leading eye centers and had reached the pinnacle of his professional career. But Ruiz was not ready to stand aside—not yet. The move to the new building represented the culmination of everything he had worked for during his career, but the morning would bring more patients to see and new issues to resolve.

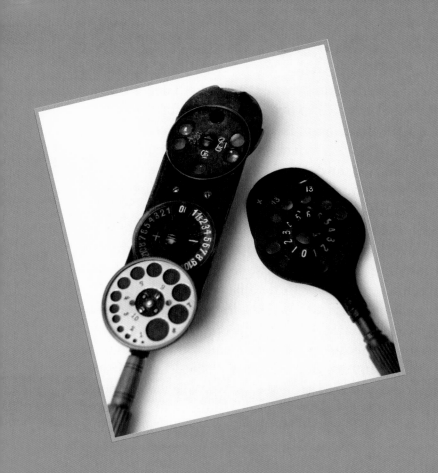

Passing the Baton

"I am relinquishing the chairmanship
of the Department of Ophthalmology.
It is time to pass the baton."

—Richard S. Ruiz, MD, July 15, 2008.

E ARLY IN 2008, after several anxious years of searching for just the right person to succeed him, Dick Ruiz finally felt that the time was right for him to step down as chair of the Department of Ophthalmology and Visual Science. Ruiz's tenure as chair was both historic in its longevity and significant in its accomplishments. During his thirty-seven years as founding chair of the department, Ruiz successfully brought together the eye service at Hermann Hospital, his private clinical practice, and the ophthalmology department of The University of Texas Medical School at Houston to create a unique model for patient care, teaching, and research. His legacy as chair would be both an inspiration and a challenge to those who would follow in his footsteps.

Throughout the years that he served as chair, Ruiz exhibited remarkable determination and an unwavering sense of purpose that enabled him to build the ophthalmology department from scratch while continuing to find new opportunities to enhance its academic and research capabilities. During this time, he successfully navigated the political minefields of academe, and, with great tenacity and skill, kept alive his dream of developing an exceptional eye center despite having to confront a host of challenges. His sense of determination and perseverance continued through the years, emerging whenever the opportunity presented itself. Prime examples of this were when he deftly seized the moment to bring the Sensory Sciences Center (SSC) back into the ophthalmology department, and then parlayed the SSC's research potential into grant proposals that brought the prestigious National Eye Institute Vision Core Grant to the department. His remarkable fundraising expertise enhanced the capabilities of the department when he utilized the Hermann Eye Fund to create matching funds that brought in additional millions of dollars in research grants and endowment funds. Learning to identify talented individuals assisted him in recruiting some of the finest researchers, educators, physicians, and staff for the ophthalmology department and for the various components of the Eye Center. Although he had stepped on a few toes over the years—as is the case with most academic department chairs—Dick Ruiz had earned the respect of his colleagues and the medical students and interns who had enjoyed the unique opportunity of training in ophthalmology at UT–Houston. Under his leadership, the ophthalmology department successfully aspired to reach the highest levels of excellence in teaching and to develop a sterling reputation in research. But after nearly forty years of hard work, the time had come for Dick Ruiz to pass the baton to a new generation of leadership.

Following the announcement that he would step down as department chair, The University of Texas Health Science Center and President James Willerson honored Dr. Ruiz with a retirement reception and program on July 15, 2008. While this event was a milestone for Ruiz, it also signaled the end of an era for the Department of Ophthalmology and Visual Science. The occasion, however, marked new beginnings as well. Following his retirement as chair, the department formally would become the Richard S. Ruiz, MD, Department of Ophthalmology and Visual

Science, and after a months-long search for a successor to Ruiz, The University of Texas would appoint Robert M. Feldman, MD as the new department chairman. Ruiz planned to continue teaching in the Medical School and treating eye patients, but now he would have more time to devote to his many outside interests and to managing the Hermann Eye Fund.

In addition to a host of family and friends, numerous colleagues, students, and well-wishers attended the reception to congratulate Ruiz and to celebrate his remarkable career and many accomplishments as department chair. A number of dignitaries also attended the meeting, conducted by James Willerson, MD, as president of The University of Texas Health Science Center at Houston. Also attending were Dan Wolterman, president and CEO of the Memorial Hermann Health Care System; UT regent James D. Dannenbaum; and a number of prominent civic leaders and members of the Texas Medical Center, the UT Health Science Center, and the Medical School. Guest speakers included Cheves M. Smythe, MD, the first dean of the Medical School; Juanita Romans, CEO of Memorial Hermann Hospital–TMC; Dan Jones, MD, chair of the Department of Ophthalmology at Baylor College of Medicine; former UT Medical School–Houston deans Drs. John Ribble, L. Maximilian Buja, and Stanley Schultz; and the new dean, Giuseppe Colasurdo, MD.

It is worthwhile to note some of the comments from that occasion in order to fully grasp the significance of Ruiz's contributions as the founding chair of the ophthalmology department and the unique role it played within the Eye Center. "This is a bittersweet occasion," said James Willerson in his opening remarks. "But the sweet part of it is that we get to congratulate, admire, and show our respect and great affection for Dick Ruiz and his family, for his leadership of the Department of Ophthalmology at our medical school, and also at Memorial Hermann." Willerson noted Ruiz's lengthy service at both Hermann Hospital and the Medical School and stated, "It would be hard to find a similar example anywhere in the world." [1]

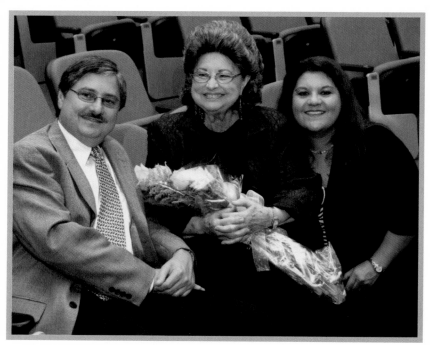

Robert Ruiz, Yvonne Ruiz, and Cindy Ruiz Kepfer.

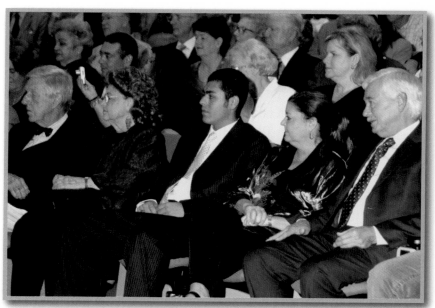

Cheves M. Smythe, Ruiz family and guests at Ruiz retirement program.

Cheves M. Smythe followed Willerson to the podium. He began his remarks by saying, "If we were in a civic environment instead of academic, I think it would be very appropriate that we start with the quote from an epitaph in St. Paul's Cathedral in London by Christopher Wren, and that is, 'If you seek his monument, look around.'" Smythe noted that the basis for the success of the Eye Center was that Ruiz "sets invariably very high standards at everything," and that providing excellent care for each of his patients always was his first priority. Dan Jones spoke next about Ruiz's contributions to ophthalmology, calling him a "Renaissance Man" and the "Dean of American Chairs of Ophthalmology." He expressed his appreciation for how Ruiz fostered collaboration between Baylor College of Medicine and The University of Texas Medical School at Houston. As a tribute, Juanita Romans presented Ruiz with a collage depicting his life in photographs. "If I look at the things that impress me most about Dr. Ruiz," said Romans, "it is that he has great passion for being a clinician and he cares about people. And you can see that in everything that he does." Romans called Ruiz a "cornerstone" of Hermann Hospital and acknowledged that in both good times and bad he had "always been there for us." Clearly, Ruiz had garnered immense respect, admiration, and appreciation from his colleagues over the years.

After brief reflections and congratulatory comments from the former deans, the Medical School's current dean, Giuseppe Colasurdo, presented Ruiz with a traditional UT retirement gift: a beautiful oak chair emblazoned with the crest of The University of Texas. Then, Colasurdo formally announced that the Department of Ophthalmology and Visual Science henceforth would be named the Richard S. Ruiz, MD, Department of Ophthalmology and Visual Science. Following Colasurdo with closing remarks, James Willerson said

> I think there is one thing that has not been said quite enough
> yet, and that has to do with your loyalty and your passion for

those things you believe in.... But your loyalty for this medical
school and for the Hermann Hospital and the Memorial
Hermann Hospital, for the Medical Center, and for those
who are here that you believe are doing worthwhile things,
is extraordinary. I am not sure I have ever met anybody who
exceeds you in loyalty and passion for people that you care
about and believe in.

Willerson then presented a bouquet of yellow roses to Ruiz's wife,
Yvonne, and a "very special gift" to Dick—a bronzed sculpture
of a Texas longhorn—remarking, "This is given to you tonight,
Richard S. Ruiz, MD, with appreciation, respect, and gratitude
for all that you have done for The University of Texas Health Science Center at Houston."[2]

Ruiz then stepped up to the podium to make a few remarks.
He thanked Willerson for organizing the reception and briefly reflected on his career. "You know, my father was a physician," Ruiz
began. "Back in those days, they called them general practitioners. But my father always said that medicine was the noblest profession. And as a young kid I watched the respect, appreciation,
and the love that the patients had for him. I never wanted to be
anything else but a doctor. I never thought of anything else." Ruiz
talked about his love for ophthalmology, for his patients, and for
Hermann Hospital. "I interned at Hermann in 1957, as Dr. Willerson said, and I immediately fell in love with that hospital. It had
an extra dimension and that dimension was the teaching—the
training programs. So, I always knew I was going to come back to
Houston and I always knew that I was going to come back to practice at Hermann." Wanting to emphasize the significance of The
University of Texas Medical School at Houston, Ruiz discussed
how it brought "many other dimensions for me in my practice
and what I wanted to do with my life." He spoke of his love for
teaching, saying that he found inspiration from "the exposure to
intelligent, highly motivated individuals pursuing excellence."
He clearly relished his leadership role in developing the Depart-

ment of Ophthalmology, expressing his gratitude for being able "to do it more or less with free rein." Following Ruiz's remarks, the audience gave him a warm, rousing, standing ovation.

Ruiz had been thinking about retiring as chair for several years, but there were many issues and complications that he felt compelled to resolve before the time was right for him to step down. He had spent most of his professional life building the Eye Center and cared deeply about its academic component, the Department of Ophthalmology and Visual Science. He thought long and hard about finding just the right person to succeed him as chair: someone who embraced the concept of the Eye Center, who understood how the various components worked in concert, and who appreciated its success. In fact, Ruiz first began to consider the ramifications of his retirement as department chair in the months before he decided to leave Houston Eye Associates. His concern that succeeding chairs would find their ability to act on behalf of the department entangled in the HEA organizational structure was the principle reason he left that group. In 1999 he named Dr. Robert M. Feldman as deputy chair of the department. Although Ruiz respected Feldman's ability, for some time he considered whether Feldman was the right person to succeed him as chairman, viewing him as "a brash young man—brilliant, but brash."

During the next nine years, Ruiz had ample opportunity to work with and observe Feldman in action. "As the years passed, I became more and more appreciative of his talents," said Ruiz. Over time he saw that Feldman possessed the qualities and the mix of talents to become a good chair. Ruiz observed that Feldman was very entrepreneurial, loved teaching and clinical research, and also demonstrated that he was loyal to the mission of the Eye Center and not looking for a department chair position somewhere else. Robert Feldman, with his exceptional training, credentials, and sterling reputation, easily could have been a candidate for department chair at any number of medical schools, and Ruiz greatly appreciated his loyalty to the Eye Center and to

UT. Although Ruiz was confident about his decision to endorse Bob Feldman as his personal choice for department chair, with several "loose ends" remaining, including the relocation of the eye clinic to the Memorial Hermann Medical Plaza, he believed that it was not yet prudent for him to retire.[3]

Several months after the move from the Jones Pavilion into the Memorial Hermann Medical Plaza, Ruiz arranged a meeting with the dean of the Medical School to discuss his retirement as chair of the ophthalmology department. Although Ruiz was confident that Feldman would measure up handily in the formal search process, recent personnel changes brought two new people into key administrative positions—Giuseppe Colasurdo as dean of the Medical School and Larry R. Kaiser as president of UTHSC–H—either of whom conceivably could have rejected his recommendation for Feldman to succeed him as department chair. Ruiz always had enjoyed good relations with the leadership at UTHSC and the Medical School, but at this time he had not become well-acquainted with either President Kaiser or Dean Colasurdo, and thus, proceeded carefully to ensure that there would be no misunderstandings that might derail his wish for Feldman to succeed him.[4]

During his meeting with Colasurdo, Ruiz told the dean of his plans to retire as chair of the Department of Ophthalmology and Visual Science. He stated that his personal choice to succeed him as chair was Dr. Robert Feldman. But the fact that Ruiz endorsed Bob Feldman as his successor did not in any way assure that Feldman would be the candidate chosen by the Medical School's search committee. Ruiz highlighted Feldman's qualifications for Colasurdo, noting that he had excellent academic credentials and possessed all the requisite skills to run the department. In addition, the fact that Feldman was already a highly regarded faculty member with an established medical practice meant that the Medical School would not have to spend vast sums recruiting and enticing him to make a move to Houston. Ruiz made it clear that he understood the protocols and hiring regulations that had to be followed, and he expected it might take as long as one year to complete the formal search process. Dean Colasurdo stated, however, that he thought it could be accomplished in a few months, perhaps by midsummer. Because of the unique organizational structure of the Eye Center and the integral role of the ophthalmology department within it, Ruiz emphasized that committee members should have a true understanding of how the Eye Center functioned and also an appreciation for its success. "This was the first time I had ever really had any interface with the dean," said Ruiz. "He was very personable and charming, and I was favorably impressed. He seemed to grasp the value of the things that had been done within this [ophthalmology] department, even though the approach had been different, and so I thought, 'Well, great!'"[5]

Assuming that the dean would act quickly to appoint a committee and get the formal search process underway, Ruiz was disappointed when, after two months, he had not heard of any movement regarding the process or the appointment of a search committee. Concerned that the committee selection was already taking too much time and that the dean might have been distracted from the search, Ruiz requested an appointment with Colasurdo to get an update and possibly to give the process a push. Another two weeks elapsed before the dean would meet with Ruiz. Colasurdo informed him that he had not yet appointed a search committee. Surprised at this lack of progress, Ruiz reiterated his plans to retire as chair in July and encouraged the dean to appoint a search committee to get the process moving. After a brief discussion, Colasurdo immediately telephoned Dr. Richard Andrassy, Chair of Surgery, and asked him to chair the search committee. As Ruiz later recalled, he heartily endorsed the selection of Andrassy as committee chair and also suggested for search committee members several fulltime clinical and research faculty who had good insight regarding the ophthalmology department and the Eye Center.

Notwithstanding Ruiz's urgency, things in academe tend to proceed at their own pace, regardless of circumstances. After this

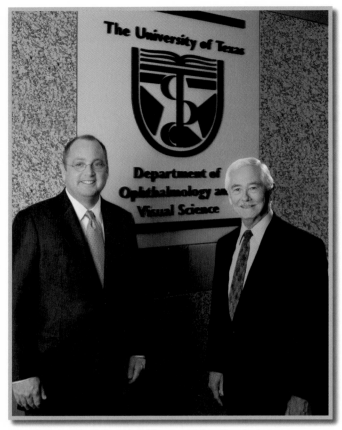

New chairman Dr. Robert M. Feldman, and founding chairman,
Dr. Richard S. Ruiz.

initial activity more time passed, and still there were no formal
announcements of a search committee and no advertisements
posted in the appropriate academic journals. Frustrated, Ruiz
called Andrassy, who replied that he was waiting for the dean to
approve the committee and set the process in motion. Finally, after another two months passed, Andrassy was able to tell Ruiz
that the committee had interviewed the candidates, that they
had been impressed with Bob Feldman, and that they had recommended him to the dean for the position. Once again, weeks
passed until, at long last, Colasurdo informed Ruiz that he had
received the committee's recommendation and he soon would be

meeting with Feldman to discuss the appointment. "But nothing formal ever happened," said Ruiz. "So, it dragged on and on."[6]

At last, in January 2009, the Board of Regents approved Feldman's appointment. The University of Texas Medical School at Houston formally announced Dr. Robert M. Feldman as the new chair of the Richard S. Ruiz, MD, Department of Ophthalmology and Visual Science. In a statement published in the Medical School's newsletter, *Scoop,* Dean Giuseppe Colasurdo stated his appreciation for Ruiz's thirty-seven years of leadership and expressed his confidence in the new chair. "I am grateful to Dr. Feldman for his recent leadership as interim chair, and I am certain that he will provide the leadership to take this department to the next level," said Colasurdo. "Please join me in welcoming him to this new administrative role and thanking Dr. Richard S. Ruiz, who has done an outstanding job as the founding chair of the department."[7]

Feldman's new job had many responsibilities, including overseeing twenty-five faculty members engaged in various educational, clinical, and research activities, along with nine residents, five fellows, and a clinical practice that treated approximately 3,000 patients per month at the Cizik Eye Clinic and Lyndon B. Johnson General Hospital. "It is a privilege to work with such a distinguished and diverse group of faculty, staff, and students," Feldman said. "Through our clinical, teaching, and research efforts, and the strong support of the Medical School and the university, we will continue to work toward advancing the national and international reputation of the department."[8]

For Ruiz, the formal announcement of Feldman's appointment came as a huge relief. "That was a critical step, because from the beginning I never wanted to create the Eye Center without it serving as The University of Texas Department of Ophthalmology, and I felt the same way about it now. I had spent my whole life—my whole professional career—creating this, and I was not about to see it turned over to somebody who could not run a hotdog stand, even though they might have a great CV." For Bob

Feldman, the formal announcement was a highly anticipated moment and also held implications for his own expectations about the future. From the beginning, he had embraced the mission of the Eye Center and fully supported Ruiz's vision of what it could be. Now, he had his opportunity to continue that legacy and to make his own mark by taking the Eye Center to an even higher level of excellence and renown: "to become the place in the region for all of our missions," said Feldman. By continuing to focus on providing the highest level of patient care, research, and education, Feldman envisioned the Eye Center attracting more residents, faculty, and financial support from a broader geographical area, further enhancing its reputation across the nation.[9]

With a new department chair in place, Dick Ruiz could focus on seeing patients, managing the Hermann Eye Fund, and taking a little more time to relax, confident that the new leadership would continue the work to which he had dedicated his life. While many challenges remained, including negotiating a service agreement with Memorial Hermann Hospital–TMC, building the endowment for the Eye Center, and the uncertain world of health care reform, Ruiz was optimistic about the future: "I think we will just get better and better as a service organization, as a teaching organization, and as a research organization."[10]

Over the years, the Eye Center has meant different things to different people. For Dr. Judianne Kellaway, teaching medical students and residents and providing care for the indigent patients were the key components that made the Eye Center so special. "We take care of people, no matter what," said Kellaway, "We never turn anybody away." Dr. Larry Brenner noted the uniqueness of the Eye Center model and the quality of patient treatment and research. "It is a vibrant place," said Brenner. "I think it has brought together the vision that Dick had to meld clinic practice and teaching and research into a compatible organization ... done a little differently than Baylor and other places."[11]

Dan Woltermann, President and CEO of Memorial Hermann Healthcare System, prepared a written statement that captured his thoughts about the blended futures of Ruiz's legacy and the Hermann healthcare system:

Memorial Hermann Healthcare System has faithfully served the Houston region for 102 years. Our system has grown from a single hospital, the Baptist Sanitarium in downtown Houston, to the largest nonprofit health system in the state of Texas. Today, the Memorial Hermann system is comprised of 14 hospitals, 57 outpatient sites, 20,000 employees, and 5,000 physicians. Our strong affiliation with The University of Texas Health Science Center—Houston has enabled Memorial Hermann to provide nationally renowned health services, such as those exemplified by ophthalmology, to all patients of southeast Texas, regardless of their ability to pay.

As we look to the future, Memorial Hermann will continue to grow to meet the ever-expanding healthcare needs of our community. This growth will be oriented towards developing outpatient services and strong clinical centers of excellence throughout the region. In order to achieve this vision, Memorial Hermann will need to create system-wide clinical services in areas such as cardiovascular, oncology, neurosciences, orthopedics, and ophthalmology. Our system-wide clinical services will be built around relationships with outstanding physicians and first-class clinical facilities.

The Hermann Eye Center/Cizik Eye Clinic is a wonderful example of how the Memorial Hermann system is achieving its vision of nationally renowned centers of excellence in clinical services. Over the years, the Hermann Eye Center has assembled a group of outstanding physicians in all sub-specialty areas of ophthalmology and combined this great clinical capability with a beautiful, state-of-the-art clinic in the new Memorial Hermann Medical Plaza. The Hermann Eye Center/Cizik Eye Clinic will be the catalyst for Memorial Hermann achieving its vision while making their services available to all in need, regardless of their ability to pay for

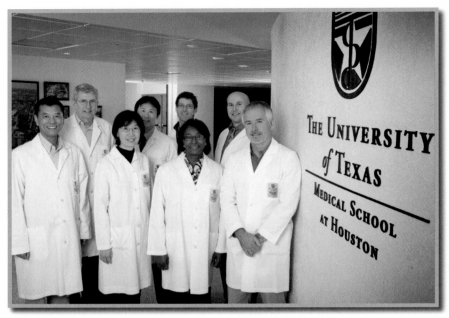

Richard S. Ruiz, MD, Department of Ophthalmology and Visual Science—Basic Science Faculty. Front row from left, Xinping C. Zhao, PhD; Alice Z. Chuang, PhD; Louvenia Carter-Dawson, PhD; and Stephen C. Massey, PhD, Director. Second row from left, Stephen L. Mills, PhD; Steven Wang, PhD; John O'Brien, PhD; and Christophe Ribelayga, PhD.

the services. The breadth and depth of ophthalmologic services provided by the Hermann Eye Center will enable our system to create the necessary centers of excellence in eye care through consolidation of services on one or more hospital campuses in the areas of retinopathy of prematurity, eye trauma, and emergencies, to name just a few. These centers of excellence in ophthalmology will be anchored at the Memorial Hermann—Texas Medical Center due to our relationship with the Hermann Eye Center/Cizik Eye Clinic and The University of Texas Health Science Center—Houston.

The Houston region has greatly benefited over many years from the exceptional ophthalmologic care provided by Hermann Eye Center/Cizik Eye Clinic's partnership with Memorial Hermann. Considering the anticipated changes that will occur in the national health care system over the next ten years, this relationship can do nothing but prosper. Memorial Hermann has been and continues to be blessed with the partnership with the Hermann Eye Center/Cizik Eye Clinic, and we look forward to developing a seamless, comprehensive center of excellence in ophthalmologic services for the community with this outstanding group of physicians.[12]

Randy Gleason, in his capacity as longtime legal counsel, first for Hermann Hospital and later for Memorial Hermann Healthcare System, often provided his legal expertise for the Hermann Eye Center and served as a board member of the Hermann Eye Fund. Gleason observed the Hermann Eye Center for most of its history, noting its critical role in providing emergency eye care for trauma patients at Memorial Hermann Hospital–TMC. "One of the things I always think about when I think about the Eye Center is that if you have an eye injury in the Houston area, Hermann really is about the only place that has eye trauma service," said Gleason. "Dick and his staff have taken care of that for decades. A lot of the patients do not have any money, and Dick and his team have taken care of those people. They have really made a huge commitment to Houston and to the Medical Center." Expressing his appreciation of Ruiz's dedication to providing a comfortable setting for patients, including his attention to the art and décor of the Eye Center, Gleason stated that Ruiz "understood that the quality of the experience is more than just having a good clinical outcome. It [requires asking,] 'How do you design an environment that the patients will feel comfortable in and that promotes confidence in the treatment?'" Gleason noted that the Hermann Eye Center offered a unique model—including the rare affiliation of a private hospital as the primary teaching hospital for a state university—that provided superior training for ophthalmology residents at the UT–Houston Medical School. "I think the UT residents in ophthalmology probably had a better learning experience than at any state university medical school anywhere in the country," said Gleason. "Dick prepared his graduating residents

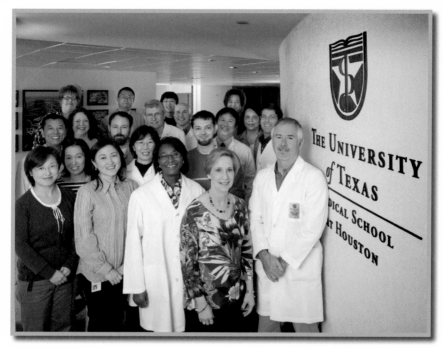

Basic Science Group Staff and Faculty.

to do private practice in ophthalmology better than any teaching program. ... they had a great university experience, but they also had a great private practice experience that [most] universities just cannot offer."[13]

This unique opportunity for ophthalmology residents was part of Ruiz's inspiration for developing a world-class eye center more than thirty years ago. The arrival of The University of Texas Medical School in 1970 and its affiliation with Hermann Hospital as its primary teaching hospital opened the door for the creation of a new model in medical education and health care. Dick Ruiz possessed the imagination and energy to seize the opportunity to bring together a private hospital, a state medical school, and a clinical ophthalmology practice in a cooperative endeavor that would create a prototype for a new era of patient care, education, and research.

Although he had stepped aside as department chair, Ruiz still had the same fire and enthusiasm for ophthalmology that he possessed when he first opened his solo practice nearly fifty years earlier. Sitting in his office on the eighteenth floor of the Memorial Hermann Medical Plaza, nearly two years after the move from the Jones Pavilion, Ruiz reflected on the future of the Eye Center. "We want to continue to do what we have been doing, and that is [to] practice superior ophthalmology; train superior ophthalmologists, teach medical students, nursing students, and technicians; render indigent care; and do basic and clinical research to try and help improve ophthalmological services for the public." As Ruiz observed, after more than thirty years, the mission of the Eye Center remained the same: patient care, teaching, and research in the field of ophthalmology.[14]

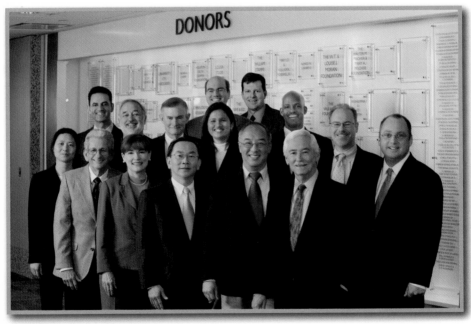

Clinical Faculty. Front from left, Nan Wang, MD, PhD; R. Larry Brenner, MD; Judianne Kellaway, MD; Richard W. Yee, MD; David A. Lee, MD; Richard S. Ruiz, MD; and Robert M. Feldman, MD. Second row from left, Reza D. Farahani, OD; Charles A. Garcia, MD; Robert W. Butner, MD; Bhavani Iyer, OD, FAAO; Garvin H. Davis, MD, MPH; Marc R. Criden, MD. Back, Nicholas P. Bell, MD and Michael C. Breckel, OD.

Ruiz faced many challenges during his career but never lost confidence in his vision for the Eye Center. He had an amazing ability to adapt to adversity and turn it to his advantage. When he saw the need for more funds to support indigent patient care and Hermann Hospital's eye service, he created the Hermann Eye Fund. When the opportunity arose to expand the hospital's ophthalmic intern and residency programs into a full-fledged academic and research environment, he seized the moment to create an Eye Center. And as sweeping changes rocked the medical world, he found ways to adapt. Now headquartered at the Robert Cizik Eye Clinic in the Memorial Hermann Medical Plaza, the Hermann Eye Center, in its partnership with The University of Texas Medical School at Houston's Richard S. Ruiz, MD, Department of Ophthalmology and Visual Science, continues as one of only two Houston institutions that provide specialty training in ophthalmology. The Hermann Eye Fund continues to fulfill Ruiz's origi-

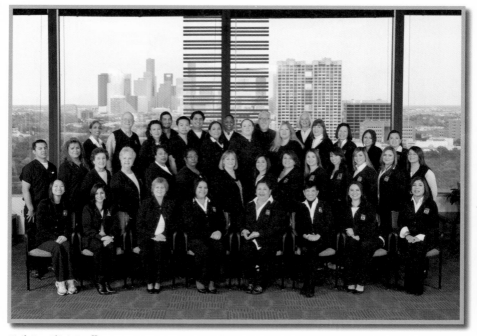

Cizik Eye Clinic Staff.

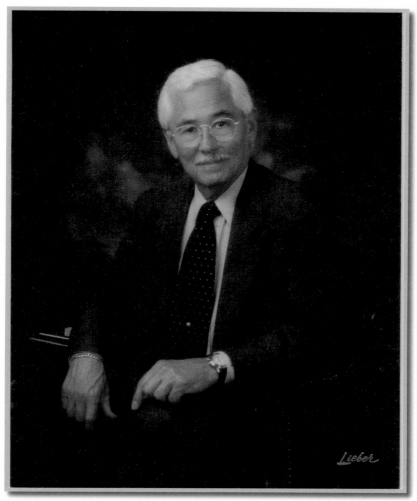

"Your best assurance of excellence in health care is having a questioning student looking over your doctor's shoulder."—Richard Stranahan Ruiz, MD.

nal aspirations by providing financial support for basic science research in the Medical School. Since it was first established, the Eye Fund has created thirteen endowments in the Department of Ophthalmology and Visual Science, including two endowments of $2 million each: the Richard S. Ruiz Distinguished University Chair and the John S. Dunn Distinguished University Chair. The John S. Dunn Chair was the first distinguished university chair established in The University of Texas System. The Eye Fund also continues to fulfill its legacy of service to the needy by providing nearly $1 million per year in services to indigent and semi-indigent patients.

The Hermann Eye Center/Cizik Eye Clinic has a long history of providing the highest level of patient care, education, and research. The Eye Center has steadfastly maintained the high standards of excellence set by its founder and remains focused on fulfilling its mission. In doing this, the Hermann Eye Center has blazed a new trail by creating a unique model for medical education and in the process, helped enhance the reputations of Memorial Hermann Hospital–TMC, The University of Texas Medical School at Houston, and the Texas Medical Center. The renowned physician and medical educator, Sir William Osler, once wrote, "The practice of medicine calls equally for the exercise of the heart and the head."[15] Perhaps inspired by his father's own example, Ruiz employed this guiding precept throughout his career and eventually assembled a team that embraced it as well. The result has been the creation of a clinical practice dedicated to providing exceptional eye care for all patients and the development of an ophthalmology department focused on training the finest eye care specialists and leading the way in visual system research.

With this proud heritage as a guide, one can only expect that the Hermann Eye Center will continue to provide the exemplary care for which it has become known, and that the Richard S. Ruiz, MD, Department of Ophthalmology and Visual Science will continue to build upon its sterling reputation in research and in training medical professionals who practice ophthalmology with compassion, exercised equally with knowledge.

Notes

CHAPTER 1

1. Abraham Flexner, *Medical Education in the United States and Canada: A Report to the Carnegie Foundation for the Advancement of Teaching* (New York: Carnegie Foundation, 1910). Interestingly, the Flexner Report concluded that of the four medical schools in Texas in 1909, "There is only one medical school in the state fit to continue in the work of training physicians. That institution is the state university; the medical school is its department at Galveston" (312). Information on the American Board of Ophthalmology available at: http://www.abop.org/about/board.asp (accessed May 1, 2008). In 1933, the American Board for Ophthalmic Examinations changed its name to the American Board of Ophthalmology. Today, it is one of twenty-four specialty boards recognized by the American Medical Association and the American Board of Medical Specialties.

2. Louis J. Marchiafava and Nancy Hadley, "The Man and His Vision: George H. Hermann," unpublished manuscript, 1992; Everett L. Goar Jr., interview by Louis J. Marchiafava, September 15, 1987. During the next few years, Goar took additional courses and training at the University of Colorado and received a doctorate in ophthalmology in 1925.

3. Marchiafava and Hadley, "The Man and His Vision;" Edward A. Blackburn Jr., "The History of the Houston Ear, Nose, and Throat Clinic," in *The Good Old Days: Memoirs of Retired Harris County Physicians*, edited by George Alexander, MD., (Austin: Sunbelt Eakin Press, 2001), 341–47.

4. The Sisters of Charity had operated St. Mary's Infirmary in Galveston since 1869 and by May 1876, had expanded into a three-story brick hospital that could provide beds for some 250 patients. Marguerite Johnston, *Houston: The Unknown City, 1836–1946* (College Station: Texas A&M University Press, 1991), 58, 96; Chester R. Burns, *Saving Lives, Training Caregivers, Making Discoveries: A Centennial History of the University of Texas Medical Branch at Galveston* (Austin: Texas State Historical Association, 2003), 9–10.

5. Ted Francis and Carole McFarland, *The Memorial Hospital System: The First Seventy-Five Years* (Houston: Larksdale Press, 1982), 5–18; Marilyn McAdams Sibley, *The Methodist Hospital of Houston: Serving the World* (Austin: Texas State Historical Association, 1989),10; Johnston, *Houston*, 139, 146–47, 181,190. Houston historian Marguerite Johnston observed that "As a railroad center, Houston had railroad hospitals that brought outstanding physicians to the city."

6. Bryant Boutwell, "Two Bachelors, a Vision and the Texas Medical Center," *Houston Review of History and Culture*, vol.2, no. 1, Fall 2004, (Houston: Center for Public History—University of Houston, Fall 2004), 8–11; Naomi S. Foster, "George H.

Hermann and History of Hermann Hospital," unpublished manuscript, 1975. Hermann's estate was valued at just over $2.6 million.

7. Foster, "George H. Hermann," 35. The three trustees were T. J. Ewing Jr., J. J. Settegast Jr., and John S. Stewart.

8. Foster, "George H. Hermann," 45–46. The committee included Dr. O. L. Norsworthy, Dr. Gavin Hamilton, Dr. J. Allen Kyle, Dr. E. L. Goar, Dr. Ron Wilson, Dr. Joseph Mueller, and Dr. R. Knox. While contractors were busy building Hermann Hospital, the new city-county hospital for the indigent opened its doors on December 2, 1924. Named in honor of the president of the Confederacy, Jefferson Davis, the new charity hospital was staffed by volunteers from the Harris County Medical Society. Early in 1925, the new Houston Negro Hospital, the gift of oilman J. S. Cullinan, opened in the Third Ward. Johnston, Houston, 242–43.

9. Johnston, Houston, 249, 251.

10. Foster, "George H. Hermann," 52–56; Johnston, Houston, 251.

11. Foster, "George H. Hermann," 57, 86.

12. Historian Louis J. Marchiafava, PhD, conducted a series of oral history interviews sponsored by Dr. Richard S. Ruiz, from 1987–89, to record the early history of Hermann Hospital.

13. Louis J. Girard, interview by Louis J. Marchiafava, September 3, 1987.

14. Elizabeth Crawford, interview by Louis J. Marchiafava, June 13, 1987; Otto L. Zanek, interview by Louis J. Marchiafava, April 8, 1987.

15. Cecil Crigler, interview by Louis J. Marchiafava, July 2, 1987. Crigler served for many years as the chair of the medical education committee at Hermann Hospital. The committee was composed of all the chiefs of the established departments: medical, surgical, and all surgical specialties. It had the responsibility for accepting interns, establishing residence quotas, and for the discipline of the teaching programs at Hermann.

16. Cecil Crigler, interview by Louis J. Marchiafava, July 2, 1987.

17. Foster, "George H. Hermann," 106; N. Don Macon, Monroe Dunaway Anderson, His Legacy: A History of the Texas Medical Center, 50th Anniversary Edition (Houston: Texas Medical Center, 1994), 137–52. See also: Frederick C. Elliott, The Birth of the Texas Medical Center: A Personal Account, edited by William Henry Kellar (College Station: Texas A&M University Press, 2003).

18. George R. Kolodny, interview by Louis J. Marchiafava, April 15, 1987.

19. Louis J. Girard, interview by Louis J. Marchiafava, September 3, 1987.

20. Elizabeth Crawford, interview by Louis J. Marchiafava, June 13, 1987.

21. George R. Kolodny, interview by Louis J. Marchiafava, April 15, 1987.

CHAPTER 2

1. Richard S. Ruiz, interview by William H. Kellar, March 22, 2007.

2. Richard S. Ruiz, interview by William H. Kellar, February 22, 2007; Chester R. Burns, Saving Lives, Training Caregivers, Making Discoveries: A Centennial History of the University of Texas Medical Branch at Galveston (Austin: Texas State Historical Association, 2003), 206.

3. Richard S. Ruiz, interview by William H. Kellar, February 22, 2007.

4. Richard S. Ruiz, interview by William H. Kellar, February 22, 2007.

5. Richard S. Ruiz, interview by William H. Kellar, March 22, 2007.

6. Richard S. Ruiz, interview by William H. Kellar, February 5, 2007; Richard S. Ruiz, interview by William H. Kellar, March 6, 2008.

7. Richard S. Ruiz, interview by William H. Kellar, February 5, 2007; March 22, 2007.

8. Shattuck W. Hartwell Jr., MD, ed., " . . . to act as a unit" The Story of the Cleveland Clinic, 2nd Edition. (Philadelphia: W. B. Saunders Company, 1985), 97, 151, 163; online at http://www.kresgeeye.org/history.html (accessed February 26, 2008). The Kresge Eye Institute became an official component of the Wayne State University School of Medicine in 1966.

9. Richard S. Ruiz, interview by William H. Kellar, March 22, 2007.

10. Richard S. Ruiz, interview by William H. Kellar, March 22, 2007.

11. Richard S. Ruiz, interview by William H. Kellar, March 22, 2007.

12. Richard S. Ruiz, interview by William H. Kellar, March 22, 2007. The five Ruiz children are Roseanna, Kathleen, Raymond, Robert, and Cynthia.

13. Dr. Ruedemann was chief of staff at Detroit Receiving Hospital and at Harper Hospital. Dr. Saul Sugar, a well known glaucoma expert, was chief of staff at Mt. Sinai Hospital.

14. Richard S. Ruiz, interview by William H. Kellar, March 22, 2007; Richard S. Ruiz, interview by William H. Kellar, March 6, 2008.

15. Arthur Gerard DeVoe, "Ramon Castroviejo, MD," Transactions of the American Ophthalmological Society, Vol. 85 (1987): 6–8. Available at: http://www.pubmedcentral.nih.gov/pagerender.fcgi?artid=1298761&pageindex=1 (accessed February 27, 2008).

16. Moorfields Eye Hospital was founded in 1805 as the London Dispensary for curing diseases of the Eye and Ear. Part of the National Health Service (NHS), the London hospital, together with the University College London (UCL), is the oldest and the largest center for eye care and research in the world. Available at http://en.wikipedia.org/wiki/Moorfields_Eye_Hospital (accessed February 27, 2008).

17. Dr. Schepens died March 28, 2006, at age 94, days after receiving the French Legion of Honor in recognition of his courageous efforts in the French Resistance during World War II. Meg Ostrum, The Surgeon and the Shepherd: Two Resistance Heroes in Vichy France (Omaha: University of Nebraska Press, 2004). Bryan Marguard, "Charles Schepens, 94, Leader in Nazi Resistance, Pioneer in Retina Surgery," Boston Globe, April 5, 2006. Available at:http://www.boston.com/news/globe/obituaries/articles/2006/04/05/charles_schepens_94_leader_in_nazi_resistance_pioneer_in_retina_surgery/); also available at www.schepens.harvard.edu; www.schepens.com and http://historywired.si.edu/object.cfm?ID=10 (accessed February 26, 2008). The Massachusetts Eye and Ear Infirmary, founded in 1824, is the second-oldest eye hospital in the United States. New York Eye and Ear Infirmary, founded in 1816, is the oldest.

18. Richard S. Ruiz, interview by William H. Kellar, March 6, 2008.

19. Richard Ruiz, interview by Louis Marchiafava, December 23, 1987; Richard S. Ruiz, interview by William H. Kellar, February 5, 2007. The group ophthalmology practice was to include Drs. Ralph Berkeley, Elizabeth Crawford, Marion Johnson, George Kolodny, and Thomas Royce.
20. Richard S. Ruiz, interview by William H. Kellar, February 5, 2007.

CHAPTER 3

1. Richard S. Ruiz, interview by William H. Kellar, March 6, 2008.
2. Royce's new group practice included Drs. Thomas Royce, George Kolodny, Marion Johnson, Elizabeth Crawford, Richard Leigh, and Ralph Berkley.
3. Richard S. Ruiz, interview by William H. Kellar, March 6, 2008.
4. Richard S. Ruiz, interview by William H. Kellar, February 5, 2007.
5. Richard S. Ruiz, interview by William H. Kellar, March 22, 2007. Ruiz recalled that Dr. Gingrich was known as "Giggles Gingrich" by the students and his faculty colleagues, due to his tendency to giggle faintly when he spoke.
6. Richard S. Ruiz, interview by William H. Kellar, April 26, 2007; March 6, 2008; Gayle Hodges, Lois Marie Dansdill Jr., interview by Louis J. Marchiafava, September 14, 1987.
7. Harry Youens, interview by Louis J. Marchiafava, July 28, 1989.
8. Richard S. Ruiz, interview by William H. Kellar, March 6, 2007. M. D. Anderson paid $60,000 per year and salary for one resident in return for complete outpatient coverage, twenty-four hour, seven-day-a-week inpatient consultation and emergency coverage, weekly ophthalmology clinics, and immediate access to all subspecialty expertise afforded by the faculty of the Department of Ophthalmology.
9. Robert Stewart, interview by Louis J. Marchiafava, August 15, 1989.
10. A. Louis Dippel, MD, and Leigh J. Crozier, MD, letter to members, active medical staff, section of ophthalmology, Hermann Hospital, January 16, 1967, Hermann Eye Center Archives.
11. Richard S. Ruiz, interview by William H. Kellar, February 5, 2007;
12. George Gilbert Pyle Jr., interview by Louis J. Marchiafava, October 31, 1987. During the late 1980s, historian Louis J. Marchiafava, PhD, conducted a series of oral history interviews with doctors and nurses who had trained or been on staff at Hermann Hospital. Many of those interviews are cited in this chapter.
13. Robert Stewart, interview by Louis J. Marchiafava, August 15, 1989.
14. Robert Lowe, interview by Louis J. Marchiafava, June 28, 1989; Sue Ellen Young, interview by Louis J. Marchiafava, September 30, 1986.
15. Charles Russo, interview by William H. Kellar, July 9, 2007.
16. Malcolm Mazow, interview by William H. Kellar, June 27, 2007.
17. Richard S. Ruiz, interview by William H. Kellar, February 5, 2007; Jeffrey D. Lanier, interview by William H. Kellar, April 15, 2008
18. Robert Lowe, interview by Louis J. Marchiafava, June 28, 1989.
19. Malcolm Mazow, interview by William H. Kellar, June 27, 2007.
20. Bryant Boutwell and John P. McGovern, *Conversation with a Medical School: The*

University of Texas-Houston Medical School, 1970–2000 (Houston: The University of Texas at Houston Health Science Center, 1999), vii; Charles LeMaistre, quoted in Boutwell and McGovern, 4–9; William S. Fields, MD, To and Through the Texas Medical Center: A Personal Odyssey (Austin: Eakin Press, 1995), 246.

21. Richard S. Ruiz, interview by William H. Kellar, March 29, 2007.

22. Bryant Boutwell and John P. McGovern, Conversation with a Medical School, 89. See also: L. Rodney Rogers, MD, "The Birth of The University of Texas Medical School in Houston," in The Good Old Days: Memoirs of Retired Harris County Physicians (Austin: Sunbelt Eakin Press, 2001), 148–67.

23. Bryant Boutwell and John P. McGovern, Conversation with a Medical School, 89–91; L. Rodney Rodgers, quoted in Boutwell and McGovern, 90–91; William S. Fields, M.D., To and Through the Texas Medical Center, 247; L. Rodney Rogers, MD, "The Birth of The University of Texas Medical School in Houston," The Good Old Days: Memoirs of Retired Harris County Physicians (Austin: Sunbelt Eakin Press, 2001), 155, 164–66.

24. Dan. G. Kadrovach, a retired U.S. Army colonel, had served as the associate hospital director since 1966 and succeeded the highly respected Dr. Leigh Crozier, who retired in October 1968.

25. Cheves M. Smythe, interview by William H. Kellar, April 13, 2007; Richard S. Ruiz, interview by William H. Kellar, March 29, 2007.

26. Richard S. Ruiz, interview by William H. Kellar, March 29, 2007; Cheves M. Smythe, interview by William H. Kellar, April 13, 2007.

27. William Fields, interview by Louis J. Marchiafava, June 9, 1989. Dr. Fields is credited with discovering the benefit of taking an aspirin a day to help prevent strokes.

28. Available at http://www.parkplazahospital.com/CWSContent/parkplazahospital/aboutUs/newsAndArticles/thehistoryofParkPlazaHospital.htm (accessed April 17, 2008); Richard S. Ruiz, interview by William H. Kellar, March 29, 2007.

29. Boutwell and McGovern, Conversations with a Medical School, 13–14.

30. Richard S. Ruiz, interview by William H. Kellar, March 29, 2007; William Fields, interview by Louis J. Marchiafava, June 9, 1989.

31. Richard S. Ruiz, interview by Louis J. Marchiafava, January 29, 1988.

32. Rice Health Facilities Studio Team, Ophthalmology Center (Rice University Department of Architecture, 1974).

33. In several documents, Ruiz made the case and highlighted the benefits of his proposal to Hermann Hospital, The University of Texas Medical School at Houston, and to his colleagues at Houston Eye Associates. See: "Proposal to Hermann," "Advantages of HEC to HH," "Advantages of HEC to UTMSH," and "Advantages of HEC to HEA," in folder "Agreement: Hermann Hospital and HEC," Hermann Eye Center Archives.

34. Richard S. Ruiz, interview by Louis J. Marchiafava, January 29, 1988; Richard S. Ruiz, interview by William H. Kellar, March 29, 2007. Richard S. Ruiz, interview by William H. Kellar, March 29, 2007; Cheves M. Smythe, interview by William H. Kellar, April 13, 2007.

CHAPTER 4

1. Minutes of the Hermann Hospital Estate Board of Trustees, April 1, 1975, 5813. The UTHSC–H had been created in 1972, under acting president Dr. John Victor Olsen, as an organizational umbrella that included all of the university's Houston medical branches except the M. D. Anderson Cancer Center.

2. William S. Fields, interview by Louis J. Marchiafava, June 9, 1989.

3. William S. Fields, MD, *To and Through the Texas Medical Center: A Personal Odyssey* (Austin: Eakin Press, 1995), 253.

4. William S. Fields, interview by Louis J. Marchiafava, June 9, 1989; Richard S. Ruiz, interview by William H. Kellar, March 29, 2007; Minutes of the Hermann Estate Board of Trustees, September 23, 1975, 5880.

5. Richard S. Ruiz, MD, Director of the Program in Ophthalmology, letter to Board of Trustees, Hermann Hospital Estate, October 3, 1975, Hermann Eye Center Archives, in folder "Agreement: Hermann Hospital and HEC."

6. Minutes of the Board of Trustees, Hermann Hospital Estate, October 21, 1975, 5886–87, in Hermann Eye Center Archive, in folder "Agreement: Hermann Hospital and HEC." This meeting apparently had been scheduled to take place on May 17, 1975 and was to have included Dan Kadrovach, Dr. Charles Berry, Acting Dean of the Medical School Dr. Robert L. Tuttle, and the chiefs of the various hospital and medical school sections, to discuss Dr. Ruiz's proposal "in order to ascertain the ramifications should Hermann accept the proposal of Dr. Ruiz." But there is no evidence that this group met, perhaps prolonging the decision on the Eye Center. See: Neill F. Amsler Jr., Executive Vice President of Hermann Estates, letter to John B. Coffee, trustee, May 14, 1975, Hermann Eye Center Archive, in folder "Agreement: Hermann Hospital and HEC."

7. Richard S. Ruiz, interview by William H. Kellar, February 5, 2007; Minutes of the Board of Trustees, Hermann Hospital Estate, December 2, 1975, 5894, Hermann Eye Center Archive, in folder "Agreement: Hermann Hospital and HEC."

8. Richard Ruiz, interview by William H. Kellar, February 5, 2007.

9. Minutes of the Board of Trustees, Hermann Hospital Estate, January 22, 1976, 5909, Hermann Eye Center Archive, in folder "Agreement: Hermann Hospital and HEC." Richard S. Ruiz, interview by William H. Kellar, February 5, 2007.

10. Rebecca Galvan, "UT Health Science Center Chief Quits Due to Animosity," *Houston Chronicle*, February 17, 1977; "The 1947 Texas City Disaster, April 16 & 17, 1947."Available at: http://www.texascity-library.org/TCDisasterExhibit/index. html and also at http://en.wikipedia.org/wiki/Texas_City_Disaster (accessed April 29, 2008).

11. Richard S. Ruiz, interview by William H. Kellar, February 5, 2007.

12. Richard S. Ruiz, interview by William H. Kellar, February 5, 2007.

13. Richard S. Ruiz, interview by William H. Kellar, February 5, 2007.

14. "HEC's Ambulatory Care Unit Integrates Specialized Area to Create a Total Eye Care Facility," *Views & Visions*, Vol. I, No. I, Fall 1977, (reprint of original), Hermann Eye Center Archive, 4–5.

15. "The Preservation of Sight and the Visual Presence of Art: A Unique Combination," *Views & Visions*, Vol. I, No. I, Fall 1977, (reprint of original), Hermann Eye Center Archive, 4.

16. Mary Jane Schier, "Center Offers Innovative Eye Care," *The Houston Post*, December 7, 1977, 4B. The Herman Eye Center held a formal opening in December 1977, in conjunction with the Congress of Ophthalmology meeting sponsored by the UT Medical School's Department of Ophthalmology. Charles Garcia, interview by William H. Kellar, August 28, 2007. Charles Garcia earned his bachelor's degree at the University of Florida and later completed medical school at Tulane in 1969. He did his internship and residency at Hermann Hospital, and completed a fellowship at Baylor College of Medicine in cornea and infectious diseases.

17. "Houston Delta Gamma Foundation Provides a Counseling Service, Volunteers, and Equipment," *Views & Visions*, Vol. I, No. I, Fall 1977, (reprint of original), Hermann Eye Center Archive, 6; Sue McRaney, interview by William H. Kellar, September 10, 2007. Sue McRaney was born on a farm in Spring Hill, Mississippi. She earned a bachelor's degree in sociology at Millsaps College in Jackson, Mississippi, and a master's degree in social work at Tulane. She was a social worker for the Orleans Parish Schools in New Orleans, and then moved to Houston in 1973. In Houston she did volunteer work and in 1977, and joined the Delta Gamma Alumni Association to work part-time as a social worker with newly blind and blind children in the new Hermann Eye Center.

18. "Hermann Eye Center Goals and Concepts: A Guide to the Future," *Views & Visions*, Vo. I, No. I, Fall 1977, (reprint of original), Hermann Eye Center Archive, 2–3; 6–7.

19. Richard S. Ruiz, MD, letter to William F. Smith, Executive Director, Hermann Hospital, August 16, 1977, Hermann Eye Center Archive, in folder "Agreement: Hermann Hospital and HEC."

20. "Hospitalized Patients Are now Part of the Team," *Views & Visions*, Vol. I, No. 2, Spring/Summer 1979, Hermann Eye Center Archive, 1–6.

21. "Hospitalized Patients Are now Part of the Team," *Views & Visions*, Vol. I, No. 2, Spring/Summer 1979, Hermann Eye Center Archive, 1–6.

22. Richard S. Ruiz, MD, letter to Neill F. Amsler, October 4, 1978, Hermann Eye Center Archive, in folder "Agreement: Hermann Hospital and HEC"; "Hermann Eye Center Sets the Pace," *Views & Visions*, Vol. 3, No. 1, Spring/Summer 1980, 7.

23. Charles Russo, interview by William H. Kellar, July 9, 2007.

24. Robert Wilkins, interview by William H. Kellar, April 22, 2008.

25. In fact, it was Dick Ruiz who first suggested the need for a free-standing, outpatient surgery facility with ample parking, to compete with other hospitals.

26. Richard S. Ruiz, interview by William H. Kellar, March 29, 2007.

27. Richard S. Ruiz, interview by William H. Kellar, March 22, 2007; Charles Garcia, interview by William H. Kellar, August 28, 2007; Robert Wilkins, interview by William H. Kellar, April 22, 2008. .

28. Richard S. Ruiz, interview by William H. Kellar, March 29, 2007; Jeffrey Lanier, interview by William H. Kellar, April 15, 2008; Robert Wilkins, interview by William H. Kellar, April 22, 2008.

29. Charles Russo, interview by William H. Kellar, July 9, 2007; Malcolm Mazow, interview by William H. Kellar, June 27, 2007.

CHAPTER 5

1. Richard S. Ruiz, interview by William H. Kellar, March 29, 2007.

2. Richard S. Ruiz, interview by William H. Kellar, March 29, 2007. Hermann Hospital agreed to take on the staff personnel of the Eye Center as hospital employees. The hospital would bill the Eye Center, which still paid the staff salaries, on a monthly basis. The move provided a little breathing room for the Eye Center to develop its cash flow. "And that helped cash flow tremendously," said Joe Leopold. "As a result of that, we never had to borrow a nickel and it was a big help for us from the hospital." Joseph Leopold, interview by William H. Kellar, November 19, 2007.

3. Richard S. Ruiz, interview by William H. Kellar, March 29, 2007; Joseph Leopold, interview by William H. Kellar, November 19, 2007.

4. "In Memory of Glenn R. Knotts, PhD," *Views & Visions*, Spring 2003, 1–4; "Purdue University Honors Dr. Knotts," *Views & Visions*, Fall 2000, 14. In 1999, Knotts's alma mater, Purdue University, honored him as a Distinguished Alumnus. His distinguished academic career included a BS, an MS, and a PhD degree that he earned at Purdue. In addition, Knotts held an MS degree in public health from Indiana University and two honorary doctorates in recognition of his professional contributions. He served as executive director of the Hermann Eye Fund from1989 to 2003. Sadly, Glenn R. Knotts died January 12, 2003.

5. "Bernice Weingarten Distinguished Professorship in Ophthalmology." *Views & Visions*, Vol. 15, No. 1, Spring 1993, 10–11; Charles A. Garcia, interview by William H. Kellar, August 28, 2007.

6. Thomas C. Prager, interview by William H. Kellar, April 22, 2008. Dr. Prager has been instrumental in outcome studies and has published extensively on this topic and on the use of electrophysiology in ophthalmology. He created a CD-ROM for the teaching of ultrasonography, and his current research involves an interdisciplinary, multi-center study that evaluates ophthalmology continuing medical education on the Internet. Prager left the Hermann Eye Center in 2009 to establish his own diagnostic business.

7. Judianne Kellaway, interview by William H. Kellar, November 15, 2007; Ruth SoRelle, *The Quest for Excellence: Baylor College of Medicine, 1900–2000* (Houston: Baylor College of Medicine, 2000), 78; Richard S. Ruiz, interview by William H. Kellar, March 29, 2007. Kellaway was appointed assistant dean for admissions at The University of Texas Medical School at Houston July 1, 2006. She also is a clinical associate professor and Stephen A. Lasher III Professor in Ophthalmology.

8. Richard S. Ruiz, interview by William H. Kellar, March 22; March 29, 2007.

9. "Meet the New Group—H/UEA: Hermann/University Eye Associates," *Views & Visions*, Vol. 16, No. 1, Fall/Winter 1994, 6; "Distinguished Doctors," *Views & Visions*, Fall 2001, 9–10.

10. Harry Sperling, interview by William H. Kellar, November 6, 2007. Sperling earned a PhD in experimental psychology with an emphasis on neurophysiology from Columbia University.

11. Richard S. Ruiz, interview by William H. Kellar, April 2, 2009. Dr. Truman G. Blocker served as acting president of The University of Texas Health Science Center–Houston, from 1977–78. Dr. Ernst Knobil served as Dean of The University of Texas Medical School–Houston, 1981–1984.

12. Richard S. Ruiz, interview by William H. Kellar, April 2, 2009.

13. Stephen C. Massey, interview by William H. Kellar, October 15, 2007; Harry Sperling, interview by William H. Kellar, November 6, 2007; Fredi Bleeker Franks, interview by William H. Kellar, November 1, 2007.

14. Stephen C. Massey, interview by William H. Kellar, October 15, 2007; "Vision Research Consortium Established at The University of Texas–Houston Health Science Center," *Views & Visions*, Vol. 16, No. 1, Fall/Winter 1994, 4–5.

15. Stephen C. Massey, interview by William H. Kellar, October 15, 2007.

16. Phyllis Deter, "National Eye Institute Awards UT–Houston Vision Core Grant," *Views & Visions*, Vol. 16, No. 1, Fall/Winter 1994, 5; "Research to Prevent Blindness: Dianna A. Redburn, PhD—Jules and Doris Stein RPB Professor," *Views & Visions*, Vol. 17, No. 1, Winter 1995, 6–7. The other two Houston Core Grant centers were Baylor College of Medicine and the University of Houston College of Optometry.

17. Dianna Redburn moved to Memphis, Tennessee in 1996 and subsequently married. In 2009, Dianna A. (Redburn) Johnson, PhD, held several academic appointments at the University of Tennessee Health Science Center at Memphis, including professor of ophthalmology; professor of anatomy and neurobiology; adjunct professor of physiology; and associate vice chancellor of academic, faculty and student affairs. Available at http://www.eye.utmem.edu/dept/faculty/djohnson. html (accessed January 25, 2009).

18. *Views and Visions*, Vol. 17, No. I., Fall/Winter 1995, 9. By the fall of 1995, the Hermann Eye Center included Richard S. Ruiz, MD; Phil A Aitken, MD; Charles A. Garcia, MD; Robert M. Feldman, MD; Judianne Kellaway, MD; Helen A. Mintz-Hittner, MD; Thomas C. Prager, PhD; Stephen G. Slade, MD; Richard G. Urso, MD; Richard W. Yee, MD; and Steward L. Zuckerbrod, MD. "Departmental Update—Stephen C. Massey, PhD, Newly Appointed Director and Professor," *Views & Visions*, Volume 18, No. I Summer 1996, 5; Stephen C. Massey, interview by William H. Kellar, October 15, 2007. Dr. Massey is professor and Elizabeth Morford Chair at the University of Texas Medical School at Houston, Department of Ophthalmology and Visual Science. He is also the director of the Basic Science Research Center.

19. "Stephen L. Mills, PhD, receives RPB Award" *Views & Visions*, Volume 18, No. I Summer 1996, 5; "Medical Museum's Eye Exhibit to Honor Dr. Ruiz," *Views & Visions*, Vol. 16, No. 1, Fall/Winter 1994, 2; "Eyeing New Exhibit," *Views & Visions*, Volume 18, No. I Summer 1996, 2–4.

20. Bryant Boutwell, PhD, "Dr. Richard Ruiz, UT System's First Distinguished Chair," *Texas Medical Center News*, Vol. 19, No. 16, September 1, 1997; *University of Texas*

System & UT–Houston Health Science Center Present: A Tribute to Richard Ruiz, MD, VHS videotape, Hermann Eye Center Archive, September 11, 1997.

21. Walter A. Zelman, *The Changing Health Care Marketplace: Private Ventures, Public Interests* (San Francisco: Jossey-Bass Publishers, 1996), 92. See also Zelman's discussion of 1990s hospital mergers, 91–100.

22. Ted Francis and Carole McFarland, *The Memorial Hospital System: The First Seventy-Five Years* (Houston: Larksdale Press, 1982), 139–140, 159.

23. Bill Mintz, "Big Merger of Houston Hospitals: Memorial Healthcare to Join with Hermann," *Houston Chronicle,* July 1, 1997, Section A, 1; "Memorial, Hermann Complete Merger," *Houston Chronicle,* November 5, 1997, Business Section, 2.

24. Richard S. Ruiz, interview by William H. Kellar, May 10, 2007.

25. Robert M. Feldman, interview by William H. Kellar, December 6, 2007; "Distinguished Doctors," *Views & Visions,* Fall 2001, 6.

26. "Hermann LADARVision® Center," *Views & Visions,* Fall 2000, 4–6; Richard W. Yee, interview by William H. Kellar, December 11, 2007. Available at http://www.ladarvision.com/ladarvision/ladarvision.asp (accessed May 31, 2008). For information on Health and Human Services CLIA program, see http://www.cms.hhs.gov/clia/ (accessed May 15, 2008).

27. Larry Brenner, interview by William H. Kellar, April 21, 2008. Larry Brenner was born in South Dakota, attended the University of Houston and the UH College of Optometry, then decided to attend medical school at UTMB. Brenner did his internship at the old Memorial Hospital in downtown Houston, his residency at the Baskin-Palmer Eye Institute at the University of Miami School of Medicine, and then returned to Texas in 1969 and opened what became a thriving ophthalmology practice in Pasadena. During the next thirty years, Brenner was very involved in state and local ophthalmology organizations, including the Texas Ophthalmological Association, where he served in a variety of leadership roles. He retired in 1999 and in March 2000, joined the Hermann Eye Center.

28. NOAA website, http://www.srh.noaa.gov/hgx/projects/allison01/synopsis.htm (accessed June 1, 2007); Alexis Grant and Lori Rodriguez, "5 Years after Allison, Is City Safer from Flooding?," *Houston Chronicle,* June 5, 2006; Dale Lezon, "Power Failures Force Hospitals to Scramble," *Houston Chronicle,* June 11, 2001; Richard S. Ruiz, interview by William H. Kellar, May 10, 2007; Sue McRaney, interview by William H. Kellar, October 6, 2008.

29. Sue McRaney, interview by William H. Kellar, October 6, 2008.

CHAPTER 6

1. Richard S. Ruiz, interview by William H. Kellar, March 29, 2007.

2. Walter M. Mischer Jr., interview by William H. Kellar, March 24, 2009; "Massive Project Serves as Vital Piece of Medical Center Puzzle," *Houston Business Journal,* 13-B, May 3, 2007.

3. Nancy Sarnoff, "Medical Team Prescribes Tower," *Houston Business Journal,* September 27, 2002.

4. Darrin Schlegel, "Hospital System Chooses New Chief," *Houston Chronicle*, October 4, 2002.

5. "Juanita Romans Appointed New MHH CEO," *Scoop*, The University of Texas Medical School at Houston, January 10, 2003.

6. Richard S. Ruiz, interview by William H. Kellar, May 10, 2007; Walter M. Mischer Jr., interview by William H. Kellar, March 24, 2009.

7. Richard S. Ruiz, interview by William H. Kellar, March 29, 2007; May 10, 2007; Walter M. Mischer Jr., interview by William H. Kellar, March 24, 2009.

8. Richard S. Ruiz, interviews by William H. Kellar, March 29 and May 10, 2007; Walter M. Mischer Jr., interview by William H. Kellar, March 24, 2009.

9. Richard S. Ruiz, MD, letter to Dan Wolterman, May 15, 2003, Hermann Eye Center Archive; Dan Wolterman, letter to Richard Ruiz, May 29, 2003, Hermann Eye Center Archive.

10. Richard S. Ruiz, MD, memorandum to Juanita Romans, June 10, 2003, Hermann Eye Center Archive.

11. Richard S. Ruiz, MD, letter to Dan Wolterman, September 5, 2003, Hermann Eye Center Archive.

12. Richard S. Ruiz, MD, letter to Juanita Romans, March 25, 2004, Hermann Eye Center Archive.

13. Juanita R. Romans, Senior Vice President of Memorial Hermann Healthcare System and CEO of Memorial Hermann Hospital, letter to Richard S. Ruiz, MD, Chief of Ophthalmology, March 30, 2004.

14. "Ophthalmology Department to be Named for Dr. Ruiz," *Views & Visions*, Fall 2004, 6.

15. Richard S. Ruiz, interview by William H. Kellar, July 24, 2007.

16. Ruiz's loyalty to Hermann Hospital was demonstrated publicly in 1992, when he wrote an eloquent defense of the hospital after it had been criticized by a local newspaper, the *Houston Chronicle*, over the composition of its board and its care of indigent patients. See: Dr. Richard S. Ruiz, "Don't Slight Hermann Hospital's Legacy to Houston's Poor," *Houston Chronicle*, April 12, 1992, 4E.

17. Richard S. Ruiz, interview by William H. Kellar, July 24, 2007.

18. "Houston's Largest Commercial Construction Project to Break Ground," *News Releases*, Available at http://www.memorialhermann.org/newsroom/092304.htm (accessed May 9, 2008); Walter M. Mischer Jr., interview by William H. Kellar, March 24, 2009.

19. "Houston's Largest Commercial Construction Project to Break Ground," *News Releases*, Available at: http://www.memorialhermann.org/newsroom/092304.htm (accessed May 9, 2008).

20. Walter M. Mischer Jr., interview by William H. Kellar, March 24, 2009.

21. Rob Patterson, "The Making of a Med-Tropolis," *MacGraw-Hill Construction*, March 2005. Available at http://texas.construction.com/features/archive/2005/0503_feature2.asp (accessed May 9, 2008); "Massive Project Serves as Vital Piece of Medical Center puzzle, *Houston Business Journal*, 13-B, May 3, 2007.

22. *Cizik Eye Clinic, Vision for the Future*, available at http://www.hermanneyecenter.com/

donation_message.htm (accessed May 10, 2008); Hermann Eye Fund, http://
www.hermanneyecenter.com/her_eye_fund.htm (accessed November 20, 2009).

23. *Hermann Eye Center Views and Visions*, Vol. 3, No. 2, Fall/Winter 1980, 1,5; *Hermann
    Eye Center Views and Visions*, Vol. 6, No. 2, Fall/Winter 1983, 5; Richard S. Ruiz,
    interview by William H. Kellar, June 17, 2008.

24. Thomas Prager, interview by William H. Kellar, April 22, 2008.

25. Richard S. Ruiz, interview by William H. Kellar, July 24, 2007.

26. Jennifer Hart, "Largest Office Building in Texas Medical Center Debuts," *Texas
    Medical Center News*, March 15, 2007. Available at http://www.texmedctr.tmc.edu/
    root/en/TMCServices/News/2007/03–15/Largest+Office+Building+in+Texas+Me
    dical+Center+Debuts.htm (accessed May 9, 2008).

28. Sue McRaney, interview by William H. Kellar, September 10, 2007.

29. Sue McRaney, interview by William H. Kellar, September 10, 2007. Richard S.
    Ruiz, interview by William H. Kellar, July 24, 2007.

EPILOGUE

1. James T. Willerson, "Comments upon the Retirement of Richard S. Ruiz," July 15,
   2008.

2. Proceedings of the Retirement Reception for Richard S. Ruiz, July 15, 2008.

3. Richard S. Ruiz, interview by William H. Kellar, April 2, 2009; June 3, 2009.

4. On September 1, 2007, The University of Texas had appointed Giuseppe Colas-
   urdo, MD, to be dean of the UT–Houston Medical School, and on August 1, 2008,
   Larry R. Kaiser, MD, was appointed as president of The University of Texas Health
   Science Center at Houston.

5. Richard S. Ruiz, interview by William H. Kellar, June 3, 2009.

6. Richard S. Ruiz, interview by William H. Kellar, June 3, 2009.

7. M. Raine, "Feldman Named Chair of Ophthalmology," *Scoop, a Publication of The
   University of Texas Medical School at Houston*, January 8, 2009.

8. M. Raine, "Feldman Named Chair of Ophthalmology."

9. Robert M. Feldman, interview by William H. Kellar, April 2, 2009.

10. Richard S. Ruiz, interview by William H. Kellar, June 3, 2009.

11. Judianne Kellaway, interview by William H. Kellar, November 15, 2007; Larry
    Brenner, interview by William H. Kellar, April 21, 2008.

12. Dan Wolterman, President and CEO, Memorial Hermann Healthcare System,
    written statement, June 2009.

13. V. Randolph "Randy" Gleason, interview by William H. Kellar, June 1, 2009.

14. Richard S. Ruiz, interview by William H. Kellar, April 2, 2009.

15. William Osler, MD, *Aequanimitas: With Other Addresses to Medical Students, Nurses, and
    Practitioners of Medicine*, Third Edition, (New York: McGraw-Hill Inc., n.d.), 440.

A Note on Sources

The secondary literature used in this study is cited in the endnotes that appear for each chapter. Primary research materials for this history came from several major sources, including the files of the Hermann Eye Center Archives; the McGovern Historical Collections and Research Center, Houston Academy of Medicine–Texas Medical Center Library; the Houston Metropolitan Research Center, Houston Public Library; and Special Collections, M. D. Anderson Library, University of Houston.

There are two sources of oral history interviews and transcripts for this project. First are the interviews conducted from 2007 to 2009 by the author, William H. Kellar, PhD, specifically for this project. In addition, from 1987 to 1992, Dr. Richard S. Ruiz sponsored a series of oral history interviews, conducted by Louis J. Marchiafava, PhD, with twenty-eight key physicians, nurses, and in some cases, the relatives of those who played a major role in the early years of Hermann Hospital and the hospital's eye service. These interviews, many of which were conducted with persons now deceased, provided firsthand accounts of the early years of Hermann Hospital and the arrival of The University of Texas Medical School at Houston. Although many of the interviewees mentioned below are not quoted in the text, all provided important historical background information for this project.

INTERVIEWS CONDUCTED BY WILLIAM H. KELLAR

Name	Date of Interview
Larry Brenner, MD	April 21, 2008
Robert M. Feldman, MD	December 6, 2007
Fredi Bleeker Franks	November 1, 2007
Charles Garcia, MD	August 28, 2007
V. Randolph Gleason	June 1, 2009
Judianne Kellaway, MD	November 15, 2007
Jeffrey D. Lanier, MD	April 15, 2008
Joseph Leopold	November 19, 2007
Stephen C. Massey, MD	October 15, 2007
Malcolm Mazow, MD	June 27, 2007
Sue McRaney	September 10, 2007
Walter Mischer Jr.	March 24, 2009
Thomas Prager, PhD	April 22, 2008
Richard S. Ruiz, MD	February 5, 2007; February 22, 2007; March 22, 2007; March 29, 2007; April 26, 2007; May 1, 2007; May 10, 2007; May 23, 2007; July 24, 2007; March 6, 2008; June 17, 2008; April 2, 2009; June 4, 2009
Charles Russo, MD	July 9, 2007
Cheves M. Smythe, MD	April 13, 2007
Harry Sperling, PhD	October 8, 2007
Robert Wilkins, MD	April 22, 2008
Richard W. Yee, MD	December 11, 2007

INTERVIEWS CONDUCTED BY LOUIS J. MARCHIAFAVA, PhD

Name	Date of Interview
Frank Barfield, MD	June 24, 1989
Alan C. Baum, MD	August 30, 1989
Alfred L. Burden, MD	May 9, 1989
Elizabeth Crawford, MD	June 13, 1987
Cecil Crigler, MD	July 2, 1987
Louis Daily, MD	August 11, 1987
Lois Marie Dansdell Jr., RN, and Gayle Hodges, RN	September 14, 1987
William S. Fields, MD	June 9, 1989
Robert B. Gillett, MD	August 30, 1989
Louis J. Girard, MD	September 3, 1987
Everett L. Goar Jr.	September 15, 1987
John Y. Harper Jr., MD	January 1, 1988
Dale W. Hayter, MD	October 4, 1987
George R. Kolodny, MD	April 15, 1987
Richard E. Leigh, MD	July 18, 1987
Robert Lowe, MD	June 28, 1989
Robert A. Neeley, MD	August 28, 1987
Jonas Proffitt, MD	November 13, 1987
George Gilbert Pyle Jr., MD	October 31, 1987
Richard S. Ruiz, MD	December 23, 1987; January 29, 1988; August 10, 1993
Edward Smith, MD	April 9, 1987
Robert Stewart, MD	August 15, 1989
Fred Thomas, MD	September 18, 1987
Hargrove F. Wooten, MD	July 26, 1989
Harry "Tom" Youens, MD	July 28, 1989
Sue Ellen Young, MD	September 30, 1989
Otto L. Zanek, MD	April 8, 1987; January 15, 1988

Index